Study Skills for Nurses

Study Skills for Nurses

Jayne Taylor

Senior Lecturer in Nursing
The Suffolk College of Higher and Further Education
and
The Suffolk and Gt. Yarmouth College of Nursing and Midwifery
Suffolk
UK

CHAPMAN & HALL
London · Glasgow · New York · Tokyo · Melbourne · Madras

Published by Chapman & Hall, 2-6 Boundary Row, London SE1 8HN

Chapman & Hall, 2-6 Boundary Row, London SE1 8HN, UK

Blackie Academic & Professional, Wester Cleddens Road, Bishopbriggs, Glasgow G64 2NZ, UK

Chapman & Hall, 29 West 35th Street, New York NY10001, USA

Chapman & Hall Japan, Thomson Publishing Japan, Hirakawacho Nemoto Building, 6F, 1-7-11 Hirakawa-cho, Chiyoda-ku, Tokyo 102, Japan

Chapman & Hall Australia, Thomas Nelson Australia, 102 Dodds Street, South Melbourne, Victoria 3205, Australia

Chapman & Hall India, R. Seshadri, 32 Second Main Road, CIT East, Madras 600 035, India

Distributed in the USA and Canada by Singular Publishing Group Inc., 4284 41st Street, San Diego, California, 92105

First edition 1992
Reprinted 1993

© 1992 Jane Taylor

Typeset in Palatino by Acorn Bookwork, Salisbury, Wiltshire
Printed in Great Britain by St Edmundsbury Press Ltd, Bury St Edmunds, Suffolk

ISBN 0 412 44070 9   1 56593 066 5(USA)

A catalogue record for this book is available from the British Library
Library of Congress Cataloging-in-Publication Data available

9304039
LB 200

Contents

Contributors

Steve Happs MSc BSc RMN RMNH RNT
Course Leader
Common Foundation Programme
The Norfolk College of Nursing and Midwifery

Tony Shepherd BA ALA MBIM DMS
Librarian
Royal College of Nursing

Jayne Taylor BSc(hons) RGN RHV Dip N(Lond) Cert Ed.
Senior Lecturer in Nursing
The Suffolk College of Higher and Further Education
and
The Suffolk and Gt. Yarmouth College of Nursing and Midwifery
Suffolk
UK

Acknowledgements

I would like to thank the following people: Steve Happs and Tony Shepherd for their valuable contributions to this book, John Blunt for his excellent cartoons, Stewart Taylor for the numerical illustrations, the 1990 RSCN students in Norwich for their help in evaluating the original works, Lisa Field, former editor at Harper Collins, for her support and encouragement, and Richard Holloway for his guidance. My special thanks to Barbara Weller who gave me the opportunity and confidence to write. Finally, I would like to thank Stewart, Laura, Victoria and Fiona who continue to put up with the chaos and who have enabled me to be what I am.

Preface

Many students of nursing, whether they are undertaking pre-registration or post-registration courses, will have been away from a college or school environment for some time. As a profession, nursing is constantly changing and the demands on students are high in terms of the commitment needed to succeed. *Study Skills for Nurses* aims to help students of nursing cope with the academic demands of both formative and summative aspects of courses.

This book is designed to help you to get the most out of your course. It is divided into small sections, some of which can be read before you start your course and others which will be of help once your course has started. The sections are designed so that they can be used independently of the other sections.

The book was written with an appreciation of how difficult it can be to start a new course and cope with other commitments as well. Many of the hints given are founded on personal experience of trying to study and continue to do all the other things you enjoy doing. The book acknowledges that most students have families, friends, pets, hobbies and pastimes which need to be managed rather than abandoned!

Jayne Taylor

1

Organizing yourself to study

Whether you are leaving home for the first time or you are a mature student starting your nursing career, or if you are already qualified and are about to undertake a post-registration course, you will need to think about getting yourself organized to study. Modern pre- and post-registration nursing courses demand a high academic standard with many colleges of nursing offering qualifications at diploma and degree levels. Managing your time effectively to include studying is something that requires careful thought if you are to be successful in gaining the qualification you require.

Some of you may be quite used to organizing your time for study if you have just left school or have recently been on an academic course. However, if this is your first time away from home you may find there are new demands on your time such as shopping for food, cooking, washing and ironing as well as all the more pleasant demands, such as parties, the cinema, the pub, etc. You will need to set aside sufficient time for study if you are to fulfil the requirements of your course successfully. It is all too easy to fill your time up with various activities and lose sight of what you are actually hoping to achieve.

For some of you, it may have been a long time since you have had to think about organizing your time to include studying as well as all the other activities you are involved with. Most adults tend to lead full lives involving social, domestic, occupational and family-related activities. Additional time for studying doesn't necessarily mean giving up some, or all, of your other commitments but it will mean readjusting your busy schedule so that studying is not neglected. For many mature students, nursing has been a long-term personal ambition and the commitment to studying has been made after careful consideration.

It is both frustrating and disappointing if your ambitions cannot be realized because you have not thought through the implications of undertaking an academic nursing course.

This chapter offers some hints about how you can organize yourself to maximize your potential for studying. Ultimately, though, we are all individuals and will have to make our own decisions according to space, existing commitments and the amount of studying required by the course we are following. It is, however, worth thinking about your circumstances and how best to organize yourself at an early stage during the course, or ideally before the course begins, rather than waiting until you have work to do and deadlines to meet. Whilst most colleges of nursing will give you some time to settle in to your new environment, it is likely to be only a few days as most courses will require you to prepare for lectures, seminars or assignments shortly after the commencement of the course.

There are several areas that need to be considered when thinking about getting yourself organized and these are summarized in the diagram below.

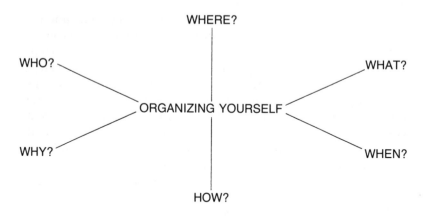

WHERE?

You will need **somewhere** to study! The venue will depend on your own circumstances, the type of study and the time you have available. The following section highlights some important considerations.

Comfort

It is important that the environment is comfortable and you are able to study in comfort. Most residences provide basic single accommodation which will include a desk and chair. If you find the chair is really uncomfortable, try using cushions either to sit on or to lean against and if that doesn't work, ask the warden of the residence if you can have a different chair.

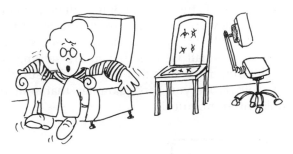

A comfortable chair is an essential commodity . . .

If you live at home you will need somewhere to work and something to sit on. It is worth trying different chairs to see which is the most comfortable – the most unlikely looking chair may be the one that best suits your needs.

Wherever you live, you should think about the environmental temperature. Try not to sit in a draught or too near a radiator (one is likely to give you a stiff neck, the other will send you to sleep!). Lighting should also be considered and it is worth investing in a study lamp, if you don't already have one.

Finally, it is important that you are able to keep yourself supplied with food and drink without having to leave your study environment every time you want a cup of coffee. Making up a vacuum flask before you start studying will keep you supplied with beverages and will prevent you losing concentration because you are thirsty. Snacks can also be prepared in advance.

Company

Most residences are designed so that each student has an individual room with use of communal cooking, bathing, laundry and recreational facilities. It should, therefore, be possible for you to study on your own if you want to.

If you live at home it may be more difficult for you to be on your own either because there is not the space or because you prefer to study whilst your family and friends are present so that you do not totally isolate yourself. It depends how easily distracted you are but earplugs are the answer for some people (a handy item if you have noisy neighbours in residence). From personal experience of studying at home with young children, I have found that they are less likely to disturb me if I am with them. A closed study or dining room door seems to attract a constant stream of small visitors! If you are settling down to study with children make sure that they are also supplied with refreshments otherwise you can guarantee that someone will want a drink within minutes!

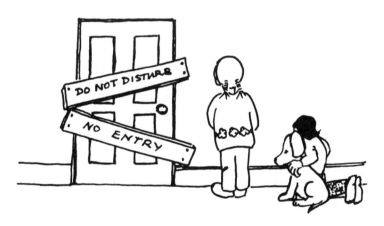

Disturbance

If you live in residence or at home there may be times when you have to say, 'please do not disturb'. A sign on the door in residence will often make friends think twice, especially if you give a time when you will be finished. Leave a pencil and paper for messages.

If you live at home, and particularly if you have children, it can be extremely difficult to arrange for undisturbed time unless you are able to work late in the evening or early in the morning. Alternatively, you can ask a trusted adult to take children off your hands for a few hours or get together with other students who are in the same position as you and childmind for each other.

It is also useful to remember that most colleges of nursing will have a library which should have a silent area where you can study in peace. It is worth considering using this facility, especially if you need to refer to literature in order to complete your studying, or if you find you are easily distracted by your environment.

Space

When you are in the full throes of studying it is useful to have somewhere to leave books open and to have journals and other material at hand. If you don't want a helpful friend to tidy them up for you then put a note on the work to say so. Likewise if you are studying in the library and go for a break, put a notice on your table to stop people disturbing your carefully sought references.

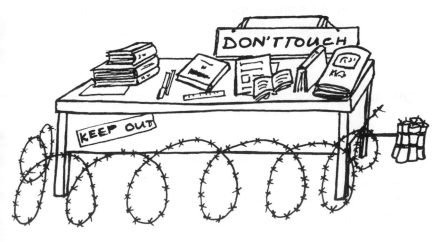

WHO?

Whether you study on your own, in pairs or in a group will vary according to the work you are doing. If you work on your own then make sure you have thought through the aspects of the environment mentioned above.

If you have to work in a group certain potential problems can occur which are worth considering. Firstly, decide on the most suitable venue and who is going to find what information. It is very frustrating to meet in someone's house only to find that no-one has brought a vital piece of reference material. Then negotiate who is going to produce what and by when. Once these targets are set they should be seen as a contract. This should ensure that everyone pulls their weight. It is very easy to get distracted and frustrated if targets are not met but at least if they have been set and agreed, all the members of the team will know who is and who is not producing the work.

If you do find you are getting frustrated with each other then it is better to discuss the situation openly rather than having a quiet moan – that doesn't help anyone! Be honest and constructively critical with each other.

When you have completed your respective parts of an assignment, it is important to sit down and 'edit' your joint work ensuring that the presentation and writing styles are similar and that you have not duplicated any information. Many group efforts have lost valuable marks because they have a 'thrown together' look, even though individuals have worked hard.

WHAT?

All nursing courses are divided into parts and each part will be assessed both formatively and summatively.

Formative assignments

Formative work which does not contribute to the overall qualifying examination of the course has several functions (English National Board (ENB) 1990):

1. It aims to maximize learning.
2. It should build on students' strengths and should enable both the student and the teacher to identify weaknesses, helping to identify individual learning needs.
3. It should encourage students to participate in self-assessment.

Formative work has to be completed and will still be assessed even though it does not contribute to your overall course marks. Formative work is vitally important in the process of the course and, because you do not risk failing the course as a result of formative work, it also allows you to use your flair and initiative. It should help you and your teacher identify areas where you need additional tutorial help.

Summative assignments

There are various assignments throughout the course which are summative assignments – that means that they are assessed and must be passed if you are to complete the course successfully. The ENB (1990) demands that colleges have clearly identified criteria relating to the conduct, content and standard of assessments. Students will usually be required to complete one part of the course successfully before they progress to subsequent parts.

Each institution will have guidelines about the number of times students can attempt summative work and it is worth finding this out before you undertake assignments or sit examinations. Depending on the institution's ruling, you will usually be given the opportunity to do remedial work with tutorial support if you fail a summative assessment. It is better, however, to seek help before assignment deadlines or sitting an examination if you feel you are having difficulties.

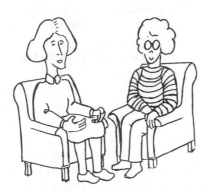

A tutorial can make all the difference.

WHEN?

When you should study very much depends on the aspects of getting organized already mentioned. If you are working with colleagues then you will need to negotiate to suit all concerned. However, individual study time can be worked in to suit your other commitments and you should aim to study when you know you are at your best. For example, some people find it impossible to work late at night and prefer to get up early and study then.

It is obviously important that you eat sensibly and get adequate rest, and relaxation and leisure times should also be worked out. Abraham Maslow (1954) proposed an interesting theory which looked at motivation and is particularly applicable here. He identified that humans have a hierarchy of needs which dominate our motives. If basic needs such as hunger and thirst are not satisfied then higher motives will not seem significant. The needs at one level must be at least partially satisfied before those at the next level become important. In practical terms, if basic needs of hunger and thirst are not satisfied, you may find it difficult to motivate yourself to pursue your intellectual interests.

If you already lead a busy life you may find that, with the additional studying, you will have to spend less time in pursuit of hobbies. Don't be tempted to give things up altogether as hobbies, especially those involving exercise, will help you to relax and reduce stress. As I know from personal experience, if you study late in the evenings it's a good idea to have a break and watch television, listen to some music or take a relaxing bath before you try to go to sleep.

The amount of time you spend studying will vary as the course goes on. The time you can spend usefully studying depends on you. You will need to get to know how long you can work without a break before you lose concentration. Some students find they work best if they have frequent breaks whilst others find that they can work for longer periods. As you get more used to studying you should be able to build up your concentration time. You may also find that if you have several areas that you need to study, it is better to spend short periods of time on each activity so that you introduce some variety into

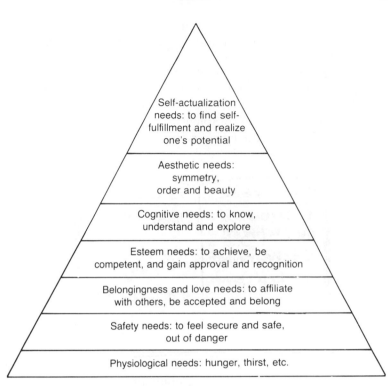

Hierarchy of motives (Maslow 1954).

your studying. If there is something you really don't want to do, try to spend a limited period of time doing it and reward yourself by doing something you find more interesting.

HOW?

Getting yourself organized and into the swing of things requires individual planning and will vary according to the demands of your course and your other commitments. However, a few suggestions are offered below. It must be stressed that these suggestions are made from personal experience of spending 12 of the last 16 years studying various nursing courses!

1. Have a notebook to write down assignments, seminars, tutorials, etc. and ensure that you record the title, guidelines

for submission, suggested word limit and date of submission as well as who you should go to if you experience any difficulties with the work.

2. Draw up a timetable for your activities each week. Start by putting in priority events (e.g. weddings, school plays, etc.) and then mark in study time. From personal experience, it always takes longer to complete assignments than you think, so add a third extra time on top of your estimated time required for study.

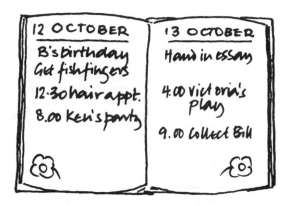

3. Set yourself targets for completion of work. If you have several pieces of work to complete over a period of time, you may find it useful to set short and long-term targets. Work towards short-term targets but gather reference material and other resources for your longer term targets.

4. If you fail to meet your own deadlines then decide what you are going to give up in order to complete the work.

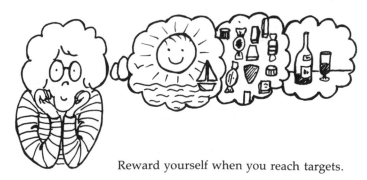

Reward yourself when you reach targets.

5. When you complete work, reward yourself (no suggestions as to how!).
6. Keep a box with index cards where you write down references and other useful information. It will save you time later on.
7. Make sure all the important people in your life are informed of your study schedule – it saves you and them becoming frustrated, irritated and hungry!

WHY?

Finally, we come to the why . . .

Students do survive courses by muddling along, leaving work until the last minute, burning the midnight oil, searching through the library to find elusive references at the eleventh hour and getting little sleep and relaxation. However, being a student is not something you should merely survive. Although you want the qualification at the end of the course, the process by which it is gained is as important as the actual product. Getting organized should be something you do for you, your friends and family. It is about getting the best out of yourself. It is about enjoying the course, meeting new people and meeting new challenges.

REFERENCES

ENB. (1990) *Regulations and Guidelines for the Approval of Institutions and Courses*. London: English National Board for Nursing, Midwifery and Health Visiting.
Maslow, A. (1954) *Motivation and Personality*. New York: Harper and Row.

FURTHER READING

Rowntree, D. (1988) *Learn How to Study*. London: Macdonald Orbis.

2

Effective use of library and information resources

TONY SHEPHERD

The ability to find and use information effectively is an essential skill for students and practitioners in a profession which is increasingly becoming more research based. This means that the results of research and good practice become widely known and accepted via journals, books and videos. Knowing how to search for sources of ideas, arguments and information, and being able to select and reject these, places the student in a strong position (Marland 1991). This chapter looks at how you can effectively and efficiently access a range of information from a variety of sources.

PLANNING YOUR INFORMATION SEARCH

Before you start looking for information you must plan, using a structured approach. This will save you time and ensure the effective use of resources. Think about your **subject** or topic and be as precise as possible. Write down the main terms or keywords covering your subject and start to list synonyms. As your search develops you will need to add extra words to these lists at different times. You can undertake **background reading** in order to help you gather keywords and synonyms – especially if the topic is new to you. General reference books such as encyclopaedias and introductory texts may be helpful, and a browse through a library's subject index can be useful.

CONSIDER THE LIMITATIONS OF YOUR SEARCH

After you have defined your subject and identified your keywords and synonyms, there are several points which you need to consider before commencing your search. These are outlined below.

1. Is your search to be in depth, covering everything available on a subject, or are you going to undertake an outline search only?
2. What period of time are you going to cover?
3. Which geographic area are you going to include? Obviously a world-wide search will be more demanding than one restricted to the United Kingdom.
4. Will you include special types of information gathered from, for example, statistical data, audio-visual records or newspaper files?
5. How much time have you available for completion of your search? Your literature searching will be reduced if your time is limited.

THE LIBRARIES AND INFORMATION SERVICES AVAILABLE

There is an ever-increasing range of information being produced in the nursing, midwifery and health visiting fields each year. No library can attempt to have everything on the subjects which you study and therefore you should be prepared to use a number of library services when searching for information resources.

You should consider using the following types of libraries but note that there are limitations as to who may use them and the range of services available. The range of libraries includes:

1. The local college or institution which you attend for the course or for tutoring sessions being provided for you.
2. The local district and/or regional library services available within the National Health Service for NHS staff.
3. University, polytechnic or other colleges. However, because of increasing student members and limited financial resources, the service on offer to 'other students' is likely to

be restricted. It is worth asking what is available and you should write or telephone first. For example, you may be able to visit a polytechnic to read a particular journal which they stock. You would not be afforded 'borrowing rights' although you may be able to pay to photocopy an article.

4. Public libraries. As a local resident you have the right to use your local public library where you should find a wide range of resources. Often these libraries have a good selection of books available on relevant subjects which may be of use to you. You can also use the interlibrary loan network available via this local library, but again you must plan ahead.

5. National libraries. Most of the Royal Colleges, professional associations and trade unions offer library and information services. You must check what is available by telephone or in writing first. If you are not a member of a college or association you should not visit them without making a prior arrangement.

Some examples of national services available are given below:

- Health Education Authority – reference use only for students.

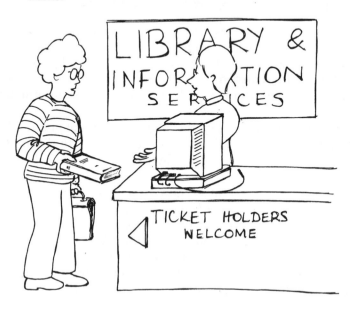

- Health Visitors Association – appointments needed.
- Royal College of Midwives – publishes a *Current Awareness Service* list.
- Royal College of Nursing – publishes *Nursing Bibliography*. Also has a large research section. Very restricted access to non-members.

Before you visit a library there are several things you should find out, which may save you time and effort. These are summarized below.

- What are the library's opening hours?
- What range of resources is available?
- Are you able to gain access to any of the available services or do you have to be a member first?
- How much professional librarian help is available?
- Do they offer an interlibrary loan system?
- Can you photocopy items?
- How much do they charge for interlibrary loans and photo-copying?

N.B. You should always start your searching at your local library.

THE INFORMATION RESOURCES AVAILABLE

A wide range of learning resources exists which you should consider utilizing for your search. Information exists in different formats and as a student and/or professional practitioner you have the opportunity to develop your skills in accessing new resources and learning how to use them effectively. The range of information resources generally available includes:

1. Printed sources – books, journals, pamphlets and theses.
2. Audio-visual sources – videos, audio cassettes, coloured slides, 'media packages'.
3. Information technology – 'local' computer databases, compact disk 'read-only memory' (CDROM) and 'on-line' terminals linked to external databases (Chapter 8). You need to think carefully about what these resources can offer you,

which of these you may need to use and how to obtain training in their use.

4. Bibliographic sources – including:
  (a) Library catalogues, printed on cards, in books, on microfiche or on computer. These catalogues list all (or most of) the resources held in the library and will usually provide:
     • an author list, which is an A–Z list of authors included in the library's stock,
     • a classified catalogue, which is a list of items arranged by subject,
     • a subject index, which lists subjects covered by the library within its classification scheme, with a code for each to allow you to locate books on the shelves.
  (b) Bibliographies, which are publications listing references to journal articles and/or books on subjects usually arranged under subject headings.

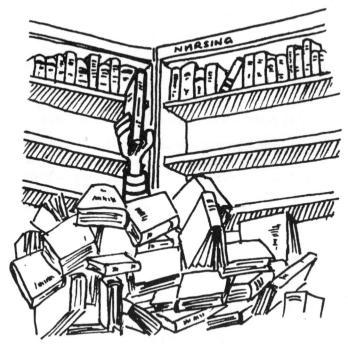

Got it!

(c) Abstracting journals, which list references to books and articles and provide, in addition, an abstract (a summary of the contents).
(d) Indexing journals, which list references in the same way as abstracting journals but without the abstract.

You should always read the 'how to use' section of these resources when you first look at them, and note how the information is arranged. Look at the contents pages and the indexes provided.

A SEARCHING STRATEGY

A number of flow charts have been produced on this topic. The diagram on page 18 amalgamates a number of these. It is, however, important to remember that if you have any doubts, you should ask the librarian for information on the most appropriate resources available and guidance on their use. Your local library could have many of the resources contained within the diagram and will almost certainly be part of a wider library service providing interlibrary loan facilities for library members. Libraries also often produce printed lists, information guides and details of available services. Such publications may include:

- journal subscription lists
- new books in stock
- how to use the CDROM.

You should look at these and if possible ask to keep a copy for future reference.

OTHER INFORMATION SOURCES

Contemporary nurses, midwives and health visitors will need to be active learners throughout their professional lives. The following examples represent sources currently available which can be useful for professional practice as well as for the information needs of students.

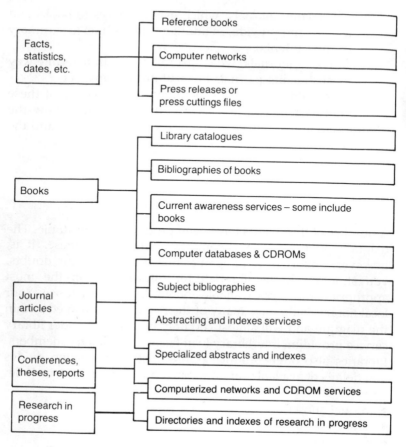

A searching strategy.

1. Directories and yearbooks, including:
   - *Hospital and Health Services Yearbook*
   - *Hospitals in the EEC*
   - *Social Services Yearbook.*
2. Reports, including:
   - The United Kingdom Central Council for Nursing, Midwifery and Health Visiting *Annual Report*
   - The Health Services Commissioner *Annual Report.*
3. Statistics, including:
   - Central Statistical Office *Annual Abstract of Statistics*

- The Department of Health *Health and Personal Social Services Statistics for England*
- The World Health Organization *World Health Statistics* (annual).
4. Guides to the literature, including:
   For periodicals, *Ulrich's International Periodical Directory* (three volumes) and *Willing's Press Guide*
   Bibliographies and periodicals indexes, including:
   (a) The *Cumulative Index to Nursing and Allied Health Literature* (1956–). This is a bi-monthly publication with an annual cumulation, known as CINAHL. Published in the USA.
   (b) The *International Nursing Index* (1966–). This is a quarterly publication with an annual cumulation, known as INI. Published in the USA.
   (c) The *Midwives Information and Resources Service* (1986–), known as MIDIRS.
   (d) The *Nursing Bibliography* (1972–). This is a monthly list of new books, reports, articles, etc. on nursing and allied subjects. Published by the Royal College of Nursing.
5. Abstracts, including:
   The *Applied Social Services Index and Abstracts* (1987–), known as ASSIA.
   The *Health Service Abstracts* (1985–). A monthly publication.
   The *Nursing Research Abstract* (1978–). A quarterly publication.

As you read through the various sources mentioned above, you should constantly refer back to your list of keywords and synonyms. It is very easy to get sidetracked when reading through information sources. You will need to convert your list of keywords so that they fit in with the keywords or subject headings which are used in the various resources. Terminology will vary, particularly in publications from overseas. Remember, also, to use the introduction, contents and index pages to discover how each source is organized. The list of subject headings is important for reviewing your identified keywords.

Finally, it may be helpful if you use small index cards, using one card per reference which enables you to rearrange your reference sources into a final reference list. Note on the back of the card where you found the reference so that you can double-check later if required.

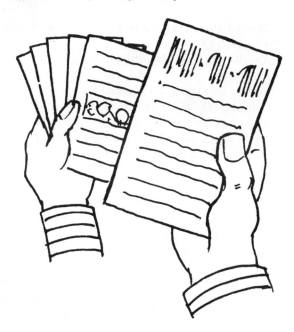

Use index cards to note references.

REFERENCING TECHNIQUES

You should keep full reference details of each book or article consulted, in order to provide academic respectability and easy transfer of knowledge in the future. Referencing is discussed in detail in Chapter 5, but briefly, if you reference a book you require the following details:

- Author(s) surname(s) plus all initials
- Year of publication
- Complete title
- Edition, if it is not the first edition
- Place of publication
- Publisher's name
- Note of series, if appropriate.

All of this information can usually be found on the front and back of the title page.

If you reference a journal article you require the following details:

- Author(s) surname(s) plus all initials
- Year of publication
- Title of article
- Name of journal
- Volume and part number of issue
- Inclusive page numbers.

All of this information can usually be found at the foot of each page, at the start of the article or on the contents page.

THE INFORMATION SEARCH PROCESS

The emphasis throughout this chapter has been on sources of information and how you can access material needed for your studies. This final section gives useful guidelines concerning the information search process.

1. As you start looking for references, it is easier to begin with recent articles and books which summarize earlier work and theories. Literature review articles are useful in that they summarize developments.
2. Having noted your references, you should obtain the articles and books which are most appropriate from the libraries available to you. Organize your references into some form of priority and check for those immediately available.

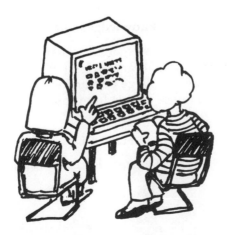

Remember, the librarians are there to help you.

3. Journal articles and books take time to arrive if you are planning to use the interlibrary loan network, so plan well ahead and allow plenty of time.
4. Keep your options open and continue to note down new references and potential sources.
5. Write down all relevant bibliographic details as well as the source of your information. This will save you time later on.
6. Remember that your local librarians are experts in finding and using information, and you should always ask for further help.

PRACTICAL TIPS ON THE EFFECTIVE USE OF LIBRARY AND INFORMATION RESOURCES

1. Clearly define your subject.
2. Decide upon your searching strategy.
3. Choose which libraries and information services are most appropriate and check if they are available to you.
4. Decide which sources of information are most suitable for your needs.
5. Begin your search, remembering to include full bibliographic details and record the source of your information.
6. Obtain books, articles and other information.
7. Read through all your gathered information and discard that which is not appropriate.

Acknowledgement

The author has based parts of this chapter upon a booklet (available from the RCN library): RCN (1988) *How to Find Information*. London: Royal College of Nursing. The author is grateful for permission to use details from this booklet.

REFERENCE

Marland, M. (1991) Skills of independence. *The Education Guardian*, 20 October, 20.

3

Effective reading and note taking

Throughout the course you will need to read a great deal of material – some of which will be useful and some which will not. It is, however, very frustrating to read every last word of a document or book and then discover that it is not useful. This is especially true if you have a lot of material to go through and only a limited amount of time in which to read it.

Another equally frustrating problem is when you 'read' a document through only to find that you have not been taking in what is written. This loss of concentration seems to occur more when we are tired but also tends to happen when the text is particularly difficult or tedious. Learning to be selective about what to read, learning to read quickly *and* being able to comprehend what is written are therefore important aspects of effective studying. This section looks at how students can develop a strategy for effective reading.

PRIORITIZING READING MATERIAL

You may find that at times during your course, you are expected to do so much reading that you do not know where to start. Most teachers will suggest reading material as a supplement to lectures and you may be required to read literature in order to complete assignments. From personal experience, I have found that it is often just not possible to read absolutely everything that is recommended and that the answer is to be selective and prioritize reading.

The first step is to clarify with the teacher which reading material is essential and what is only recommended. If you have a particularly heavy study schedule this will enable you to select the important texts which you know you must read.

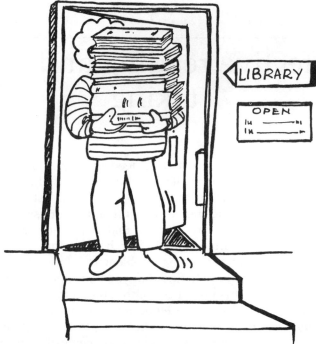

There is likely to be a lot of reading.

Secondly, you need to consult your notebook containing details of work to be completed and identify dates by which reading must be completed. This should help you to prioritize reading and set deadlines for reading each text.

Finally, when you have the chance but before the deadline for completing reading, take time to look at recommended reading and note down the content of the text. You can do this very easily by taking brief notes from the abstract or summary in the case of a journal article, or from the index or contents page in the case of a book.

EFFECTIVE READING

There may be times when you are given set or essential texts to read and you therefore have little choice but to sit down and read them. It is always a good idea to have pen and paper handy to make notes or, if the text is your own, you may prefer to use a highlighter pen to emphasize key points. Be careful not to overuse highlighter – I've seen many journal articles and books that have more highlighted sections than plain text. It is also unwise to highlight books or articles that you may use in the future for another purpose. It can be very frustrating to find a book that highlights the bits you are no longer interested in!

One system for effective reading is the SQ3R system which is described below (SQ3R stands for Survey, Question, Read, Recall and Review).

1. Survey

When you first pick up your text, do not be tempted to write anything until you have looked through or surveyed the whole text. It is always useful to start with the abstract or contents page/index. Then let your eyes run over the text, taking in headings, diagrams, tables and summarized sections. You should not read word-for-word at this stage.

2. Question

When you have finished surveying the text, sit back and reflect on what you have read and ask yourself certain questions. On your initial reading, try and put the text into the context of what you are studying. For example, if you are studying stigma in health care and are asked to read Stockwell's *The Unpopular Patient* (1974), ask yourself how the text contributes to what you have already learned and decide which points you should be looking for within Stockwell's book. Students who are studying the text in relation to stigma will need to concentrate on different aspects of the work from students who are studying it in order to identify the methodologies used for the research.

When you have reflected on what you have read, ask yourself which parts of the text you need to reread carefully and which parts you can safely resurvey. Write down your initial thoughts about important points. Finally, ask yourself if the text is really going to be helpful to you. If you decide it is, then go on to the next stage.

3. Read

The second time you go through the text, read more slowly but only read word-for-word the sentences or sections that are necessary to your work. If you cannot understand words then take time to look them up. Write the definitions down so that you do not forget meanings (self-adhesive notes are ideal for this purpose). Check that you are understanding what is written – most of us, at some time, have read something and have not taken in a word of it. Think carefully about the text and go back again to sentences that are confusing. If the sentence is long or contains, for example, double negatives, break it down into small parts to try and make sense of it. If you still find you cannot understand then make a note to ask your subject teacher for help.

4. Recall

When you have reread and resurveyed appropriate sections of the text, it is important that you again reflect on what you have read and put it into the context of what you are studying. This is important because the next stage involves making notes and you need to be absolutely clear that you have understood the text. If you have not understood it there is the danger that your notes will be inaccurate and will not reflect the text.

How often you stop to reflect will depend on your ability to concentrate and the nature of the text. Most books and articles, however, are written so that there are obvious stopping points. During the recall stage, summarize in brief note form the main points highlighted in the text and decide if there are areas you have not understood. Try rereading confusing sections and go back to your brief notes to see if it now makes sense.

5. Review

Reviewing is the most important stage of SQ3R, because it helps to clarify ideas and ensures that you have not missed important points in the text. Reviewing involves going quickly through the survey, question, read and recall process a second time – preferably after a break. It may seem tedious but is almost always worthwhile. If you have the time, it is better to leave the review for at least a day after reading. However, an hour or two is sufficient to be able to benefit from the last stage of the reading process.

NOTE TAKING FROM TEXTS

When you have read your text it may be appropriate to take notes either for future reference or for immediate use. If it is an article or book that you are going to keep, then notes can take the form of key headings and the appropriate page. If it is something you cannot keep, your notes will need to be more comprehensive. There are three stages to making notes from a written text.

Firstly, you should write down your own interpretation of what you have read. This will help you to remember what information you gathered and why it was important to you.

Secondly, you should carefully detail important facts that may help you to remember the text. Write down main headings and important points as well as any related ideas. If you are taking notes in order to write an essay, you may wish to include some idea of when the information will be useful (introduction, section A, conclusion, etc.).

Finally, write down other salient information and/or quotations which you may need to refer to, with the appropriate page number. It is useful if you are reading a government report, for example, to write down the terms of reference or, if you are reading a research report, to write down the aims of the study. If you know you cannot keep the book or article, remember to note the full reference.

A useful idea is to keep a box of index cards which indicate the article and key points. File these cards under subject headings so that you build up your own resource box for future reference.

NOTE TAKING FROM LECTURES

Taking notes from a lecture serves three main purposes. Notes will help you to recall the lecture in future, will help you to clarify the material discussed during the lecture, and can aid your concentration. Note taking from lectures involves different skills from note taking from reading material. Some lecturers make it very easy to take notes whereas others will not give you time to ask for clarification of points or to take useful notes. It is important that you ascertain if there are 'handouts' before you start to take notes. It is frustrating, to say the least, to spend time during a lecture taking careful notes only to be told at the end that the information is on a handout. You may also ask the lecturer – if you are not told – if you may ask questions during the lecture or if you should wait until the end.

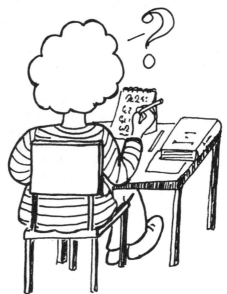

Careful note taking will prevent confusion later on.

When taking notes it is useful to develop your own short-hand. Miss out superfluous words such as 'the', 'and', 'but', etc. Try to be consistent with your abbreviations and shorthand. It may be months or years before you refer to some notes again and it is very frustrating if you cannot understand your own notes.

If you miss a word or cannot understand something during the lecture then leave a dash and ask the lecturer to explain at the end. It is also a good idea to leave a margin as you can jot down related references and asterisk (*) those things that the lecturer tells you are important. Read through your notes as soon as possible after the session, and if necessary rewrite your notes to ensure that you have understood all the points. It will also help to reinforce what has been said in the lecture. If the lecture is one of a series by the same teacher, it is useful to read through your notes before the next session so that you can clarify with the lecturer confusing points arising from the previous lecture.

There are many ways of taking notes and it is worth experimenting to see which way suits your needs. The most usual three formats are summary, framework, and pattern.

1. Summary notes

Summary notes involve writing down, in a condensed form, the content of the lecture. The problem with this form of note taking is that you can become so intent on writing that you fail to listen and assimilate information effectively. In the past, as a way of trying to keep awake in exceptionally uninteresting lectures, I have made accurate summary notes. Unfortunately, I have little recollection of the actual lectures!

2. Framework notes

Framework notes are more difficult to make but are much less demanding in terms of concentration and time, and are far easier to understand when you review them in the future.

Frameworking involves the use of letters, numbers, boxes, lists and diagrams. Main themes are underlined and subthemes are numbered. At the end of the lecture, go back and label main

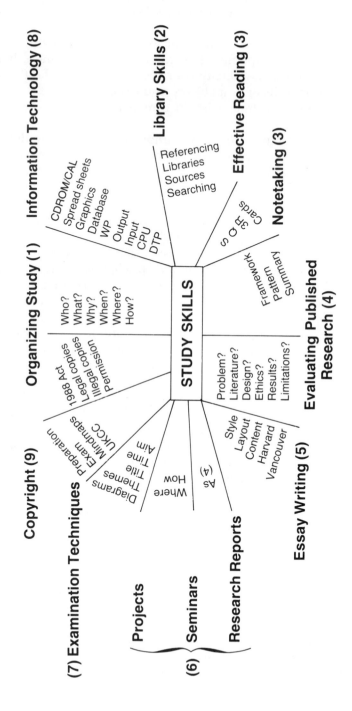

Patterning from a centre theme.

themes with letters, i.e. theme A, theme B, etc. The most important notes from the lecture can be boxed, in order to accentuate their importance.

3. Pattern notes

Patterning is usually only possible if you are familiar with the way the teacher delivers a lecture. The ideal type of session is where the teacher starts with an overall topic heading and then expands. The topic would therefore be the core and the related points would branch out from the centre (see facing page). Patterning can also be linear (see below). Pattern notes are extremely useful for revision as they are easy to remember and follow logical thought patterns.

EFFECTIVE READING AND NOTE TAKING

essential recommended — ask lecturer

1. Prioritizing reading material – reading lists – assignment dates

dictionary

survey question read recall review

2. Effective reading – SQ3R – highlighter

relevant? why?   headings where?   salient points quotations terms of reference aims cards

3. Note taking from texts – first impressions – facts – other information

summary pattern linear framework   handout?   asterisk re-write

4. Note taking from lectures – recall – clarify – concentrate – shorthand

Pattern lines.

If you leave space between each note it will enable you to add related points or references later.

STORING NOTES

Taking notes will be a waste of time if you never refer to them again. Their main purpose is to help you during the course, but unless they are systematically filed you can waste valuable time trying to find them. Ring binders are still one of the most effective ways of filing notes and they are relatively inexpensive and easily stored. It is worth buying a separate binder for each major subject you are studying. Use dividing cards to separate subthemes within subject areas. It is better if you file notes as soon as possible after making them. I find it useful to stick a piece of lined paper on the inside of each ring binder to write down the contents. It can save time later on.

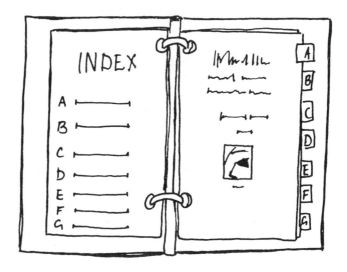

PRACTICAL TIPS ON NOTE TAKING

1. If the teacher displays points on an overhead projector, it usually means those points are important so note them down. N.B. Some teachers are prone to overusing the overhead projector, in which case the above point will not apply!

2. Always write down references and quotations (with page numbers if known). This will enable you to find out more information if you want to clarify points or widen your knowledge.
3. Make notes of any part of the lecture that is accentuated or appears to be particularly important.
4. Always read through notes as soon as possible after a lecture. If the lecturer is a regular teacher, clarify confusing points at the earliest opportunity. If the lecturer is a guest speaker, ask the usual subject teacher or your personal tutor to clarify points for you.

Exercise

Try making summary, framework and pattern notes from a chapter in one of your course books. Decide which form of notes would be easier to remember, for instance for an exam, and which form enables you to reproduce the text accurately (try writing prose from your notes in a week or two).

REFERENCE

Stockwell, F. (1974) *The Unpopular Patient*. London: Royal College of Nursing.

FURTHER READING

Buzan, T. (1989) *Use Your Head* (3rd edition). London: BBC Books.
Rowntree, D. (1988) *Learn How to Study*. London: Macdonald Orbis.

4

Evaluating published research

Nursing has been striving to become a research-based profession for many years. The profession has been criticized in the past for the lack of research undertaken and for persisting in traditional practices which in many instances are of no value to patient care (Walsh and Ford 1989). Over the last 20 years more nurses have undertaken research. However, utilization of research by practising nurses has been limited in many areas. There are three major reasons for this:

1. Researchers tend to shroud their research in academic 'jargonese' (Hockey 1987).
2. Nurses do not read research.
3. Nurses do not have the skills to be able to evaluate research effectively.

This chapter looks at how to read and evaluate published research. This is a skill that is necessary for several reasons.

1. You may be asked, as part of an assignment, to evaluate research.
2. If you undertake research as part of your course, evaluating other people's research will help you to clarify the direction of your own area of enquiry.
3. It will prepare you for using research in a practical way, to improve the quality of nursing care.

Reading and evaluating research does require you to have some knowledge of research methodology and many pre- and post-registration courses include research appreciation within the curriculum. However, there are different levels of evaluation and it is possible to assess some of the strengths and limitations of research by following a simple format. It is suggested, however, that before you start to evaluate research you ensure that you have a research methodology text (e.g. *Primer of Nursing Research* (Castles 1987) or *Essentials of Nursing Research* (Polit and Hungler 1989)) available for reference.

READING RESEARCH

When you have gathered one or more pieces of research you should first of all decide whether it is going to be useful to you. The process of SQ3R (Chapter 3) may help you decide. It will also familiarize you with the style of the researcher and the content and layout of the study.

If you decide that the research is useful there is a series of questions which you should attempt to answer. Have a notebook and pencil so that you can write down the relevant answers.

Introduction and the problem studied

Researchers will usually 'set the scene' for their enquiry by defining the problem that led them to undertake the research and giving a rationale for the study. Ask yourself if the problem seems important. Some researchers will outline the purpose of their enquiry, research questions, objectives and/or a hypothesis within this introductory section. It is, however, more usual for these to be detailed following the literature review, as one of the main purposes of searching the literature is to enable the researcher to refine their ideas and increase knowledge of the subject being studied.

Literature review

All research studies should review other research and literature which relates to their identified problem. Reviewing literature identifies what research has already been done in a particular field and helps to shape the researcher's ideas. When reading a literature review as part of a research study, you need to ask several questions:

1. Is the literature relevant to the study?
2. How old is the literature? If it is old, does it matter?
3. Does the researcher use literature from one country or from many countries. Does it matter?
4. Is the literature described or does the researcher attempt to review each piece of literature and discuss its strengths and weaknesses in relation to the other literature reviewed?
5. Does the researcher discuss the implications of the literature?
6. Are the sources of the literature used clearly documented?

Research questions, objectives and hypotheses

Following the literature review and before the methodology section of the research report, the researcher should clearly identify the purpose of the study. This may involve the identification of a number of questions which they wish to answer or objectives which they set out to achieve. As a result of the questions or objectives, a hypothesis may or may not be formulated. A hypothesis is a statement which the researcher sets out to either support or reject. An example is given below:

A ward sister may identify that student nurses who work more than seven days without a day off tend to have an increase in sickness. The aim of her research may be to discover if working seven days or more without a break

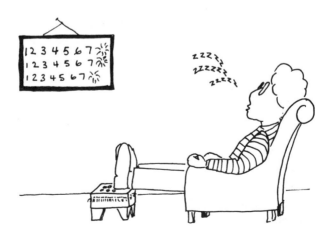

increases sickness rates. She could express this as a question which could be: 'Do student nurses who work more than seven days without a break have an increased sickness rate?'. Alternatively the sister could turn her question into a hypothesis or statement, which could be: 'Student nurses who work seven days or more without a break have increased sickness'.

The use of questions and/or hypotheses depends upon how the sister decides to investigate the problem. This is discussed more fully later in the chapter.

Sample

When the researcher starts to plan research, decisions have to be made about how the problem is to be investigated and how many people or subjects need to be involved in order to achieve the aims of the research. The researcher should state how many people or subjects were involved and how they were chosen to participate in the study. Some researchers will study an entire population (the total number of people who could potentially be included) and others will study a sample proportion of the population. If the subjects within a defined sample refuse to participate the researcher should refer to the number(s) of such subjects involved, and similarly if subjects withdraw after the study is under way. If the researcher used a questionnaire, the response rate should be clearly stated.

If a sample is used you need to decide if the people within the sample are representative of the total potential population.

An example is given below:

If a college of nursing wished to undertake a study of student sickness rates at hospital X, the total population would be the total number of students in training at hospital X. If there were 200 students, the researcher could decide that rather than include everyone, a proportion of the total should be studied. How that proportion is chosen is vitally important to the study. The researcher could choose a sample of 50 students at random, so that every student has an equal chance of being included in the study. If the choice is random, the sample should be representative of the population and implications drawn from the results can be applied to the total student population. If, however, the researcher's sample only included 50 first-year students, their sickness patterns may not be representative of second and third-year student sickness patterns. The implications of the study could not therefore be applied to second and third years.

If the researcher is undertaking an experiment, which usually involves manipulation of one group of subjects and comparing the effects of the manipulation against a second unmanipulated group known as the **control group**, it is important to ascertain how the researcher assigned subjects to each group. A further example is given below:

> If a researcher decided to set up an experiment to look at the effects of night duty on sickness rates, it would be necessary to compare sickness of students doing night duty with those doing day duty. The two groups of students should be similar and the only definable difference should be that one group does night duty and one group does not. Ideally, the students should be at the same stage of training and their assignment to the night duty or day duty groups should be at random, so that each student has an equal chance of being placed in either group. If, for example, the researcher compared first-year students who only do day duty with third-year students who do night duty, the results could be attributed to reasons other than the manipulation (in this case, night duty).

Ethical considerations

Research involving people is governed by codes which are designed to protect them and ensure that they do not suffer physical, psychological or social harm. Researchers should always consider the ethics of their research and, if necessary, should obtain permission from appropriate bodies. Nurses undertaking research on patients must always consult the ethics committee, and should state that they have done so within the study. The appropriate managers should also be consulted and their permission obtained.

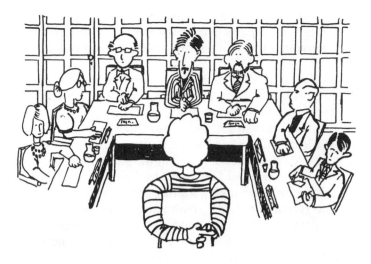

The subjects involved in research should normally have the opportunity to give their **informed consent** or to refuse to participate. Informed consent can only be given by subjects if they have received information relating to the purpose of the study, what they will be required to do if they agree to participate, and what will happen to the results of the study. They should also be informed as to whether they will be identified or if their responses will be anonymous and regarded as confidential. Details of explanations given to subjects should be clearly documented in the study.

Subjects should be allowed to withdraw their consent at any time during the enquiry.

Methodology

There are two major approaches to research: qualitative and quantitative. Most research books include discussions about both, and indicate the sorts of problems which would usually be studied quantitatively and those which would usually be studied qualitatively. Depending on the approach used, the researcher will use various **data collection instruments** in order to gather the information required to achieve the aims of the study. Data collection instruments include questionnaires, interviews, biophysical measures (e.g. thermometers, blood analysis, tape measures, etc.), observation schedules, etc. The researcher should state why a particular instrument was chosen and you should ask yourself if you feel the method used was appropriate.

The use of data collection instruments is important when evaluating research. Many researchers will use previously tried and tested instruments (such as anxiety scales, visual analogue scales, attitude measures, etc.) and they should state who designed the instrument and when it was used. If the researcher designs new data collection instrument, e.g. a questionnaire or an attitude scale, it should be tested to ensure it is reliable. This is often done by undertaking a **pilot study** which is like a trial run of the research using a small sample (usually 10% of the intended sample). If a pilot study has been undertaken, the researcher should state how this was carried out and give the results. If any changes were made as a result of the pilot study, these should be clearly stated.

Finally, it is also worth mentioning that some research will include a variety of data collection instruments, which can enhance the validity of the research.

Results of the study

The results of the study should be reported clearly and presented in a logical way. If tables, graphs or charts are used they should be easily understood and should be applicable to the study. Chapter 6 discusses appropriate ways of presenting numerical data.

Any statistical tests used to analyse data and test hypotheses should be explained and the observed values found and the level of **probability** stated. A knowledge of statistics is valuable when evaluating research in order to judge if the right statistical test has been used and if errors have been made. The Further Reading section at the end of this chapter gives useful references.

Following the results section, the researcher should discuss and interpret the findings. Results should be discussed in relation to the purpose of the research, the research questions or objectives and the hypothesis (if applicable). It is also usual to refer back to the literature review where relevant. The researcher should also highlight any limitations of the research. For example, if the response rate to a questionnaire was very low, it could have yielded atypical data which would influence the findings.

Most (but not all) research will have implications for practice and the researcher should discuss these fully. As a result of the study some researchers will also make recommendations which should relate to the results. In addition, the researcher may suggest areas where future research is needed. It should be remembered that a great deal of research actually raises more questions than it answers.

OVERALL IMPRESSIONS

Following your evaluation of research, it is always worth reflecting on the study as a whole and asking yourself a few questions.

1. Was the study readable and interesting?
2. Did it really achieve its purpose?
3. Did it include any irrelevant information?
4. Does it contribute to existing knowledge?

PRACTICAL TIPS ON EVALUATING RESEARCH

1. Read the research study through, following the SQ3R system before you start to evaluate it formally.
2. Design a numerical coding system for undertaking your evaluation. Published research (especially when it is presented as a précis) can appear muddled and may not follow a logical format. Using a code can clarify the points for you. For example, label problems as (1), literature review as (2), research questions/objectives as (3), and so on.
3. If you are comparing the results of two or more studies, use different coloured highlighter pens to accentuate related points. For example, if study A discussed the beneficial effects of using dressing X on leg ulcers, study B found dressing X made no significant difference and study C found that dressing X delayed healing, highlight them all in the same colour so that when you come to write about dressing X

you can easily find the appropriate sections in all three studies.
4. Remember that even if a piece of research is not useful for a particular assignment, it may be relevant in the future. Make up a card with the full reference and a brief description of the study and file it.

REFERENCES

Hockey, L. (1987) Issues in the communication of nursing research. *Recent Advances in Nursing*, **18**: 154–67.
Walsh, M. and Ford, P. (1989) *Nursing Rituals: Research and Rational Actions*. London: Heinemann.

FURTHER READING

Castles, M. R. (1987) *Primer of Nursing Research*, (Chapter 12). Philadelphia: W.B. Saunders Co.
Polit, D. F. and Hungler, B. P. (1989) *Essentials of Nursing Research*. Philadelphia: J. B. Lippincott Co.
Walsh, A. (1990) *Statistics for the Social Sciences*. New York: Harper and Row.

5

Essay writing and referencing

Most people have had to write essays at some time during their lives, but fully referenced, research-based, academic essays can present difficulties for many students. This chapter looks at how to write academic essays and accurately reference your work. The information given here aims to help you with your essay writing but you should always check the guidelines for each assignment with your teacher for the precise requirements.

ESSAY WRITING

Essay writing is never easy and can be extremely time-consuming. The content of an essay is what will gain you the majority of your marks but the presentation of the material will help to create a favourable impression and will assist the teacher to assess your understanding and interpretation of a subject. With badly presented work, there is also the danger that the teacher will not actually be able to read or interpret what has been written, so marks will undoubtedly be lost. It is worth checking with the teacher who will be assessing your work what percentage of marks, if any, will be assigned for presentation. Whilst you should always aim to hand in carefully written work, a knowledge of how marks are weighted will help you to know what the teacher is expecting.

The following section looks at how to lay out essays and discusses content and style of academic prose.

Layout

There are several things you can do to ensure your essay is correctly set out. Essays should always contain an introduction, a 'middle bit' and a conclusion. They may or may not make recommendations. Content is discussed in the next section.

Before you start to write your essay you should check with your teacher the following points:

- Does the essay have to be typed or can you write it out? If typed, are there any stipulations about spacing, e.g. double spacing?
- Can you write on both sides of the paper?
- What referencing style should you use?
- What information should you include on the title page, e.g. name or examination number, date, institution?
- Do you need to leave margins on one or both sides of the pages?
- Any other guidelines?

In addition to these points there are several basic things you can do to make your work more aesthetically pleasing.

1. *Quotations* If you need to quote directly from a published work it looks neater if the quote is slightly indented. You should always start on a new line when you begin the quotation and recommence text on a new line. The text should be quoted verbatim and the page number included. For example:

> Buzan (1989) discusses that the brain is able to sort information which is non-linear, a point which has recently been confirmed by other research:
>> 'Each area of research is discovering to its amazement and restrained delight that the brain is not only non-linear but is so complex and interlinked that it guarantees centuries of exhilarating research and exploration.' (p93)
> In practical terms the brain can sort such information as photographs . . .

2. *Diagrams* If you include diagrams, tables or graphs you should allow adequate room so that they do not appear to be cluttered. Diagrams should be clearly labelled and should appear with relevant portions of text. For further information on this, see Chapter 6.

Content

Most of the essays you are asked to write will involve studying the literature and writing about it. The flow chart below outlines the process of organizing your essay writing:

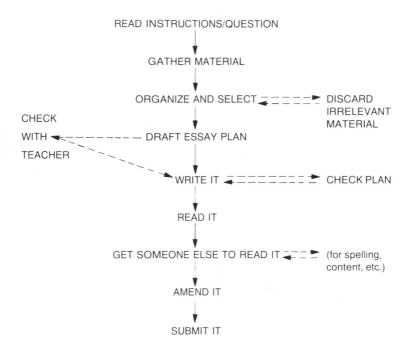

The first stage is to gather literature and other material from appropriate sources (Chapter 2 gives information on literature searching). Read through literature as you obtain it and make notes about which section of the essay it will be appropriate for. Highlighter pen can be useful for marking relevant parts of the text. Discard material which will not be used but if you feel it may be appropriate at a later stage, make up an index card with the bibliographic details and a summary of the material.

The next stage is to draft an essay plan which should be checked, if possible, with your teacher, or if not with a colleague. When you have done this, you can start to write your essay. It is a good idea to write each paragraph on a separate sheet of paper at this stage so that you can add in further information if necessary. It is always difficult to calculate your wordage so separating paragraphs will enable you to identify areas where you can add or subtract words.

After you have written your first draft, read it and ask someone else to read it. I always ask a teacher or colleague to read work at this stage, and my long-suffering husband. You then have the benefit of someone who is able to judge the content as well as someone who can correct grammar and flow. Make any necessary amendments on your rough draft and reread it. It is sometimes useful to read it out loud and record it on tape. You will soon pick up repetitive words and sentences as well as confusing passages.

The final stage is to write it for submission. If you are writing it out by hand, you will need to allow plenty of time – it will take you longer than you think. Have some white paper eraser handy and write in black ink so that you can make a photocopy of your work. Teachers have been known to lose assignments!

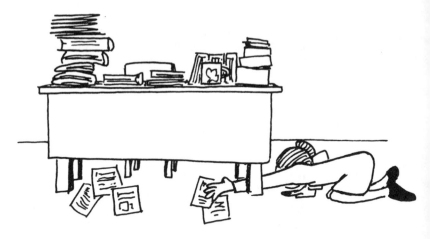

If you are required to have essays typed throughout your course it is worth enquiring if the college has word processors for students' use. Word processors save time, especially when it comes to amending text, and many of them also check spelling and count words. If someone else is typing your work, allow yourself time to read it through and have it amended if necessary.

It has already been mentioned that essays should have an introduction, a middle bit and a conclusion. The following section outlines the principles of what you should include in which bit.

1. *The introduction* This should give an overview of the subject and outline the points that you are going to discuss in your essay. It is often useful to start your essay by restating the question in the form of a statement and then take the major areas for discussion from the wording of the statement. Do not include in your introduction things that are irrelevant or that you are not going to expand on.

You may feel you wish to rationalize your approach to the subject and it may be appropriate to define certain issues. For example, if you are writing an essay about health education you might give a definition of what health education is.

2. *The 'middle bit'* This is where you discuss the main themes that you have already mentioned in the introduction. There may be one theme that has different aspects to it or there may be several themes. If you can, allow your 'middle bit' to develop logically and link areas if possible. It is usual to start with general issues and progress to more specific areas. If there is only one theme, the general issues would be discussed in early paragraphs and more specific issues later. If there are several themes and each theme takes the form of a paragraph, the beginning sentences should be general with more specific information closing the paragraph.

3. *The conclusion* Here, you pull your work to a close. It should contain the major points in a summarized form and refer back to the original question. In addition, as a result of the essay, you may be asked to make recommendations. Do not, however, make recommendations about things that you have not discussed. Your conclusion should not introduce any new ideas but you may highlight areas that you feel need further study. It is always worth making it clear when your conclusion is beginning. One way of doing this is to start your conclusion with, *To conclude . . .*

Style

Many students find it difficult to write essays in an academic style and it takes practice and discipline to produce work which is not 'journalistic'. Some assessors will allow students to write in the first person but many will not. With thought, you can write in the third person without too much difficulty. Two examples are given below, the first written in the first person and second written in the third person:

Example 1
During this essay I will discuss three factors which can influence health. The factors I have chosen are diet, smoking and sexuality.

Example 2
During this essay three factors which can influence health are discussed. These factors are diet, smoking and sexuality.

Another common problem with style is the use of sexist language (Eichler 1988). This is apparent in four forms:

1. Using male terms for generic purposes, e.g. man is a complex being.
2. Use of non-parallel terms, e.g. a man and his wife.
3. Consistently naming one sex before another, e.g. he/she.
4. Using generic terms when referring to one sex, e.g. referring to parents when only discussing mothers.

As with eliminating first person terminology, getting rid of sexist language is not usually difficult. Two further examples are given below; the first includes sexist language and the second does not.

Example 1
During the admission interview the nurse should ensure that she allows time for the patient to ask questions. If the patient is confused it may be necessary to ask one of his/her relatives to confirm details.

Example 2
During the admission interview the nurse should allow time for the patient to ask questions. If the patient is confused it may be necessary to ask a relative to confirm details.

REFERENCING

Referencing work correctly is vitally important as it tells the assessor where you have found your information, how up to date it is, and if it is appropriate to your essay. If necessary, it enables them to go to the source of your information to read the work at first hand. It also helps the assessor to differentiate between your personal thoughts and experiences and those of others.

There are two basic styles of referencing, described below, although you will find variations in some journals and text-books. Both styles are acceptable academically; however, you should not mix styles. Some colleges will specify the use of one particular style and individual teachers may express a preference. You will need to check before you start to write your assignment.

The Vancouver style

The Vancouver style is also referred to as the numerical system. The *Nursing Times*, for example, uses this system and it involves the use of numbers within the text which are cross-referenced at the end of the essay. For example:

Children should be accompanied by their parents when they stay in hospital[1,2] although it is generally thought that as they get older they are better able to deal with their experiences[3,4].

References[1,2], etc. are given in full in the reference list as follows:

1. Jones, J. (1990) Children in hospital. *Nursing Times*, **85** (15): 14.
2. Blake, D. (1985) Teenagers in care. *Nursing Standard*, **2** (3): 12.

If you refer to the reference by Jones more than once during the essay, it will always be [1]. For example:

> Two studies on children in hospital by Harris [11] and Jones [1] have looked at the need to prepare children prior to their admission . . .

or

> Two studies on children in hospital [11,1] have looked at the need to prepare children prior to their admission . . .

Cited works

The above examples show the uncomplicated use of the Vancouver system. There are, however, instances when it is not quite so simple. For example, if you have used a book by Muller, Harris, Wattley and Taylor which refers to a study by Hawthorn, you should reference it as follows:

> A study by Hawthorn [5] looked at the nursing care of children in hospital.

The reference list would give the reference of the book by Muller *et al.* as:

5. Muller D., Harris P., Wattley L. and Taylor J. (1992) *Nursing Children. Psychology Research and Practice*. London: Chapman & Hall.

It would not in the above instance be appropriate to reference the Hawthorn study directly because you are discussing what Muller *et al.* have written about Hawthorn's work, not your own interpretation of it.

(Where there are more than two authors, it is usual to use the first author's name followed by *et al.*)

Edited works

Many books are written by a group of authors, who contribute individual chapters, with an overall editor. This can pose problems if you are referring to a chapter within an edited book. The usual format is to refer to the chapter author in the text but to refer to the book editor and title in the reference list. For example:

Writing on health promotion in adolescence, Taylor [6] discusses the need for health education material to be age appropriate.

The reference would be set out as follows:

6. Taylor, J. (1992) Helping the sick and well adolescent. In Webb, P. (ed.) *Health Promotion and Patient Education*. London: Chapman & Hall.

The Harvard style

The Harvard style again indicates the source of information within the text but instead of using numbers, the author's surname and the year of publication are given and the full reference is included at the end of the work. For example:

Children in hospital should spend time with their parents (Smith 1990). Hawthorn (1975) advocated this idea and it has since been reiterated by other researchers in this field (Rowe 1990; Wells 1987).

At the end of the work references are then organized into alphabetical order as follows:

Hawthorn, P. (1975) *Nurse, I want my mummy*. London: RCN.
Rowe, J. (1990) No place like home. *Nursing Times*, 89 (4): 14–15.
Smith, S. (1990) *Children in Hospital*. London: Hodder and Stoughton.
Wells, R. (1987) Staying in hospital. *Nursing*, 15 (6): 23–5.

Cited works

As with the Vancouver system, there are complications when you wish to mention an author whose work is referred to in a journal article or book but you do not have a copy of the original work. The work would be referred to as follows:

A recent study by Smith (in Walsh and Ford 1989) suggests that many traditional forms of ointments used on wounds were harmful.

In the reference list you would refer only to the work of Walsh and Ford:

Walsh, M. and Ford, P. (1989) *Nursing Rituals: Research and Rational Actions*. London: Heinemann.

Edited works

As with the Vancouver system, edited works can cause problems. If you were referring to a chapter written by an author in an edited work using the Harvard system, it would be as follows:

Taylor (1992) discusses the role of the teacher as a health educator.

In the reference list it would be listed as follows:

Taylor, J. (1992) Helping the sick and well adolescent. In Webb, P. (ed.) *Health Promotion and Patient Education*. London: Chapman & Hall.

These two referencing styles are relatively simple and are usually used in a standardized way. It is, however, worthwhile checking with your teacher if you have any problems. Further suggested reading is given at the end of this chapter.

One final point. **References** are those works which are actually mentioned in your essay. A **bibliography** is a list of further material which has not been directly mentioned by you, but which has given you background information and may have influenced your work. A combined list may under certain circumstances be acceptable but it is always best to find out what is required before submitting the work.

PRACTICAL TIPS ON REFERENCING

1. If there are more than two authors you can use *et al.* in the text but you should always write the names of all authors as they appear on the cover of a book or at the heading of a journal article in the reference list. If there are two authors, both names should appear in the text and in the reference list.

2. If you reference a book, you should always include the place of publication and the publisher in addition to the author(s), date of publication and title.

3. If you reference a journal article, you should include the volume number and the part number (if there is one) of the issue from which the article came. It is not usually acceptable to write the date of the issue in a reference list. You should also include inclusive page numbers when you reference journal articles, as well as the author(s), year, the title of the article and the journal title.

4. If you reference a book, you should underline the title of the book. If you reference a journal you should underline the journal title (e.g. Nursing Times). You don't need to under-line chapter titles in edited works.

5. Many books are reprinted either in their original form or as updated editions. If the book has been reprinted but not published as a subsequent edition, the first date of publica-tion is the date you reference. However, if the book has appeared as a new edition (suggesting that the text has been updated and amended) you should reference the edition you have used. For example, *Study Skills for Nurses* is in its first edition and is simply referenced as Taylor (1992). If it is reprinted in 1994 without changes being made to it, it should still be referenced as Taylor (1992). If, however, changes are made to the text in 1996 it will appear as a second edition and would be referenced as follows:

Taylor, J. (1996) *Study Skills for Nurses* (2nd edition). London: Chapman & Hall.

REFERENCES

Buzan, T. (1989) *Use Your Head* (3rd edition). London: BBC Books.
Eichler, M. (1988) *Non-Sexist Research Methods: A Practical Guide*. London: Allen and Unwin.

FURTHER READING

Holm, K. and Llewellyn, J. (1986) *Nursing Research for Nursing Practice*. Philadelphia: W.B. Saunders Co.

6

Projects, seminars and research reports

During your course you may be asked to present a seminar, submit a project for assessment and, on some nursing courses (usually only those validated to degree level), you may be required to undertake a small research study. This chapter looks in detail at projects, seminars and research reports and gives practical information about each. It is obviously also important to seek guidelines from the teacher who sets the assignment so that you are aware of the criteria for assessment.

PROJECTS

The term **project** can take on many different meanings so if you are asked to undertake one you need to clarify exactly what is expected of you. A project usually takes the form of an extended essay with supporting diagrams and tables. These can be used to give visual impact to support written information and also as a way of presenting statistical information.

Students are usually given some choice about the exact topic for a project although some limitations may exist depending on whether it is part of the assessment for a single subject area or is part of a course. For example, as part of a sociology module you may be asked to undertake a project looking at an aspect of social class. Your exact choice of title may be left up to you. Alternatively, as part of a post-registration course you may be given a completely free choice about the topic area and will be able to choose a subject that is interesting and useful for you both personally and professionally. Remember, however, that you may be working on your chosen topic for several months, so if you start to become bored with it, you may have difficulty motivating yourself to work on it.

Whether you have limited or free choice about a project title, you should always draw up a plan which should include the following points:

1. the title;
2. the aim of the project;
3. the themes you will be looking at;
4. supporting information, e.g. diagrams, graphs, etc.;
5. your time scale.

If possible, you should ask for a tutorial so that you can check your plan and ensure that your proposed project is suitable. The teacher may also be able to give you advice about where to find information. An example of a project plan is given below:

A student on a post-registration child care course is asked to undertake a project over a six month period, with a maximum word limit of 3000 words. The student has a completely free choice of topic and decides to look at HIV infection in children because it is a topic that she finds interesting, she feels she ought to know more about it and she is aware that there is sufficient published material for her to use. Her plan is as follows:

Project title: HIV infected children – the role of the nurse.
Project aim: The project will explore the needs of HIV infected children and their families and will discuss the implications for the nurse in the hospital setting.
Themes: 1. What the human immunodeficiency virus is.
2. The historical perspective.
3. How children become HIV infected; vertical transmission, infection from blood, blood products and bone marrow, sexual transmission.
4. The natural history of HIV in children.
5. The needs of the child and family; physical needs, psychological needs, social needs.
6. The role of the nurse.
Supporting information: Diagram of the virus; graphs illustrating statistical information about the virus; diagram of a child showing potential manifestations of AIDS; case history;

nursing care plan showing physical precautions to prevent the spread of the virus in hospital.

Time scale: Month 1 – literature search to be completed and requests sent.

Month 2 – all literature and other information gathered.

Month 3 – review literature and sort according to themes.

Month 4 – write first draft. Have tutorial.

Month 5 – final draft of prose to be completed.

Month 6 – supporting information completed.

Throughout the project preparation period, journals will be checked monthly for newly published relevant material.

PRACTICAL TIPS ON PROJECT PRESENTATION

1. The project should be logically set out with headings to break up the text.
2. Diagrams and tables should be clearly labelled and should be situated with relevant text.
3. Literature used should be clearly and accurately documented. A reference list and further reading section should be included at the end of the text.
4. Any material included as appendices should be referred to within the text and included at the back of the project, after the further reading section.
5. The project should be bound according to the guidelines.
6. Pages should be numbered.
7. A title page should be included, giving the title of the project and your name, as well as other information requested in your guidelines, e.g. the date of submission, the course being followed.
8. It is useful for the reader if you include a contents page listing the main headings and subheadings used in the project. You cannot complete this until you have written the project.

For further information about the presentation of prose, see Chapter 5. Information about presenting statistical material is given later in this chapter.

SEMINARS

A seminar can be defined as a small class, organized by student(s) or teacher(s), which will promote discussion and thought about a particular topic.

A seminar can take the form of a brief formal presentation about a given topic followed by discussion, or can be totally participant-led. All those attending should be given the opportunity to put forward ideas, opinions, questions and solutions. It is advisable that all participants should come to the seminar with background knowledge and thoughts about the proposed topic.

The seminar organizer does, however, have additional responsibilities which are outlined below. These guidelines should be used in addition to those issued by the subject teacher.

Preparing the environment

There are some aspects relating to the environment that you need to consider.

The seating arrangement is important and can encourage or inhibit group participation. If the chairs of participants are behind desks with the seminar organizer at the front, the impression will be of teacher and student rather than equal participants. Chairs placed in rows will often result in those at

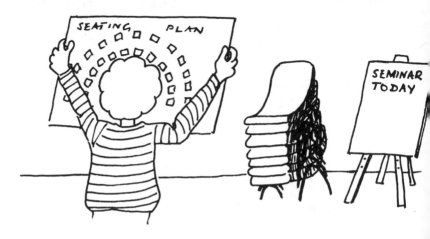

the back not being included in discussion and participants will not be able to have eye contact with each other. The most satisfactory arrangement is circular or semi-circular which emphasizes the equality of all those present. If a brief presentation is to be made, the speaker should be seated near to the audio-visual equipment, e.g. overhead projector, video recorder, etc. Other participants should be asked to move their chairs back for the presentation and close the circle during the following discussion.

Audio-visual equipment required should be checked before the seminar to ensure that it is in good working order. If a video is to be used it should be loaded into the recorder and the starting point on the video found. Slides should be loaded and the focus checked.

Initiating discussion

If the organizer intends to make a presentation in order to trigger discussion, material should be prepared in advance and should be clear and relevant to the topic area. It is sometimes useful to highlight the anticipated discussion points on an overhead projector at the start of the seminar. This gives some structure to the proceedings and can be useful if discussion relating to one topic area dries up. It is also useful for summing up and the organizer should ensure that an acetate pen is available so that unanticipated discussion topics can be added to the list. When writing on acetate, your writing should be larger than usual and you should only include key points (not more than six or eight). Try not to write too close to the edge of the acetate and use a piece of lined paper under the transparent sheet so that your writing is straight.

Clarifying language and defining terms

The seminar organizer should ensure that a dictionary and other relevant literature is available so that issues can be clarified as they arise. It is useful for participants if the organizer provides a reference list of key texts so that they can follow up points after the seminar.

Summarizing seminar content

At the end of the seminar the organizer should sum up key points.

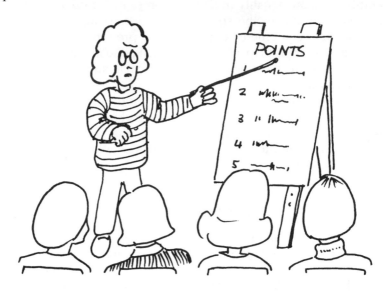

Follow up

Following the seminar the organizer should ensure that relevant information is circulated to participants. For example, if an issue was raised about which there was no information to hand, the organizer is responsible for finding the appropriate literature and circulating the reference to participants.

RESEARCH REPORTS

In some nursing courses students are required to undertake research as part of the course assessment. You should be given guidelines relating to the expected content of projects and some indication is usually made in relation to the word limit. It is not within the remit of this book to look at how to undertake research as it is assumed that you will have been taught the appropriate skills as part of your course. Many students have, however, lost valuable marks because they have incorrectly presented their research and the aim of this section is to describe one of the usual formats for writing a research report and how to present statistical information.

The title page

It is usual to start your report with a title page which should give information including your name (or examination number), the course, the college, the date of submission and the title. Your title should reflect what your report is about.

Acknowledgements

Most research reports involve other people, whether it be a statistician who has helped you to analyse your data, a friend who typed it for you or your family who have been forced to eat their meals on trays for six months because you took over the dining table! It is usual to acknowledge such help. It is, however, possible for an acknowledgement list to get out of hand so try to limit thanks to those who made essential contributions (or sacrifices!)

Contents page

The contents page should give the main themes of the study with appropriate page numbers. You may also give a list of tables.

Abstract or summary

The abstract should give a brief résumé of the study including the rationale, the broad aim(s), an outline of the sample, a brief account of the main findings and a summary of any recommendations made.

Introduction

The introduction should set the scene for the study and include information about how the study originated, why the study is being undertaken, the significance of the problem or issue being investigated, and what the research expects to contribute to existing knowledge.

The literature review

The literature review involves selecting appropriate references and providing an analytical and critical evaluation. It is usual to review literature of a general nature before that which is more specific. All literature should be relevant to the problem being studied and linked to the problem where appropriate. Any implications drawn should be clearly stated. The views of the authors whose literature is reviewed should be compared and contrasted.

A final point about literature is to remember to include classic works. Further information about literature searching is given in Chapter 2.

The purpose

After the literature review the purpose of the study should be clearly stated. This can take the form of research questions, research objectives or a research hypothesis. If there is more than one they should be placed in order of priority. Questions, objectives and hypotheses should be concise and specific.

Methodology

Firstly, the population(s) or sample(s) used for the study should be described, giving details of numbers used and the characteristics of subjects, e.g. 50 children admitted to hospital for routine minor surgical procedures or 30 nurses undertaking a post-registration degree in nursing. You should justify both the numbers used and the characteristics. Sampling techniques should be clearly defined and the type of sample stated, e.g. random sample, convenience sample, cluster sample, etc.

If questionnaires are used the response rate obtained should be stated. If the response rate is low you will need to reflect that the sample may be atypical and remember to discuss the effects within the limitations section of the study.

Secondly, the research design should be discussed with

details about how validity is to be upheld. The data collection instruments should be discussed in detail and, if appropriate, included as an appendix to the study. If a data collection instrument designed by another researcher is used, details of its use and reliability, as well as appropriate references, should be given. Details about how variables are controlled and measured should be given.

Finally, ethical considerations should be discussed and you should state what you perceive as being the major ethical issues and how you handled them. Your discussion should give details including information given to subjects, permission sought and obtained and any other related information. It should be made clear exactly what the subjects needed to do within the study.

Pilot study

It is not always necessary to carry out a pilot study. However, if you have designed your own research tools or amended those of someone else, you may need to undertake a pilot study in order to evaluate the reliability of your data collection instruments (see Polit and Hungler (1989), for a comprehensive discussion on evaluating reliability). There are certain protocols which should be followed when testing the reliability of tools and these should be described in this section. If amendments need to be made as a result of the pilot study, they should be clearly stated.

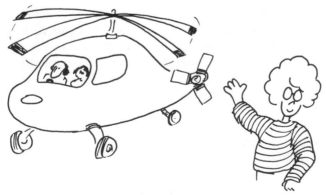

Here's a pilot, I can study him.

Results

The results of the study should be presented in a value-free way. If statistical tests are used they should be clearly explained and observed values and probability levels given. You should indicate if levels of statistical significance obtained are sufficient to reject your null hypothesis.

It is acceptable to report numbers within the text but if you start a sentence with a number you should write it in full. For example:

Forty one percent of respondents replied Yes and 59% replied No to question 4, which asked if they felt that smoking should be banned from all forms of public transport.

Information given in diagrammatic form should be clearly labelled and interspersed with relevant written text. It is rarely necessary to present data both diagrammatically and within the text but more usual to state that the results of a particular question are given in table X. Table and figure numbers should always be in sequence as they appear in the text. Further information about presenting statistical data is given in the following section.

Discussion

Following the value-free reporting of results, a discussion should be included where you can interpret your data. During your discussion you should link results back to your research questions, objectives and hypotheses. It may also be appropriate to refer back to your literature review. For example, if your findings uphold or contrast with the findings of previous research, you should discuss possible reasons for these similarities or differences.

Limitations of your research should also be discussed at this point, including failure to control or identify variables, sampling issues, reliability of data collection instruments and external validity.

Recommendations

Most research will have implications. These may include the need to change current practice or could suggest areas where further study is necessary, perhaps with a larger sample in a wider setting. A great deal of research will raise more questions than it answers and some will not have any implications at all. Try not to be disappointed if you do not achieve the results you anticipated. If you have followed the correct protocol your research will still be valuable. Some of the most interesting research I have undertaken has failed to support a hypothesis but has led to further research because of the data yielded.

Conclusion

Your conclusion should pull together the main points from your research and summarize the study. Its value in relation to change should be discussed with brief reference to noted limitations. It is usual to make a final statement linking your findings with your research questions, objectives or hypotheses.

References

A list of references should be included either in numerical order (the Vancouver style) or in alphabetical order (the Harvard style). Full details of referencing are given in Chapter 5.

Bibliography or further reading

A list of reference sources used but not cited within the text may be included after the reference list. Some colleges allow students to combine reference and bibliography lists and you should therefore seek clarification from your teacher.

Appendices

Appendices are included, if relevant, at the end of the report. Information included does not normally count towards the overall word limit of the project (check this with your teacher), and can include supporting information, models, printed extracts, data collection instruments, etc. Appendices should be numbered with roman numerals, e.g. I, II, III, IV and a list of appendices included, giving the number and content of the material.

PRESENTING STATISTICAL INFORMATION

Data can be presented in the form of tables, graphs and charts which can give added visual impact to the text, as well as reducing the wordage. The following section discusses the appropriate presentation of statistical information as an alternative to written text.

Tables

Tables are the most straightforward way of presenting statistical information and have the advantage that percentages and/or raw data can be easily seen.

It is important, however, that tables are not confusing and can be read without difficulty. Tables should only contain information that is relevant but should contain enough information for the reader to be able to understand what is being presented without needing to refer back to the text. Each table should be clearly labelled and the source of the information given if appropriate. An example is given on the facing page.

Line graphs

Line graphs are very useful for showing trends and should enable the reader to understand relevant information easily. Line graphs have an x and a y axis (the x axis is the horizontal axis). It is usual practice for frequency to be measured on the y axis. The x axis usually indicates the time scale (e.g. a year). As with tables, line graphs must be clearly labelled and particular attention should be paid to scales used. The reader should also be able to work out the exact figures from the graph so information relating to frequency scales should be clear (e.g. 1000s). Each point on the scale should be equal. An example is given on the facing page.

AGE GROUP

	under 1	1–3	4–7	8–11	over 11
Admission to Ward 4 by diagnosis in July					
Infectious diseases	14	11	7	6	4
Respiratory	26	19	11	9	9
Surgical	17	16	25	28	14
Malignant	1	2	6	7	4
Burns	2	4	1	2	1
Fracture	1	0	2	6	21
Total	61	52	52	58	53

Table of admissions to Ward 4 by diagnosis in July.

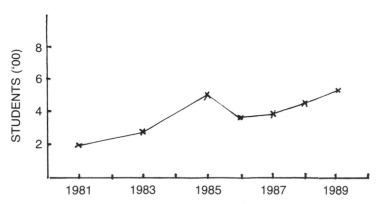

Line graph showing pass rates for students undertaking statistical evaluation between 1981–90.

Bar charts

Bar charts are ways of showing frequencies for discontinuous categories. Each chart should be clearly labelled and the reader should be able to interpret the data easily. Bar charts can be drawn either horizontally or vertically. An example is given below:

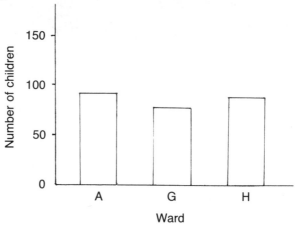

Bar chart showing admission rates of children during June 1992.

Histrograms

Histograms are bar charts that represent continuous data and are therefore useful for indicating trends. The principles of using line graphs apply to histograms. Again, each chart must be clearly labelled and scale is very important. An example is given below:

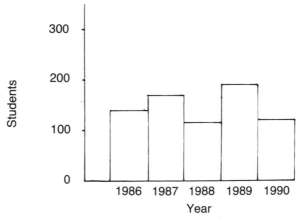

Histogram showing number of student passes in physics.

Pie charts

A pie chart is another way of presenting statistical information visually and is a circle where 360° are used to represent 100% of a sample. It is still important that the reader can work out exact figures from the information given and the charts should be labelled accurately.

One problem with pie charts is that there is a limit to the number of divisions that can be made in the pie without it becoming very difficult to interpret. The suggested maximum number of divisions is eight. An example of a pie chart is given below:

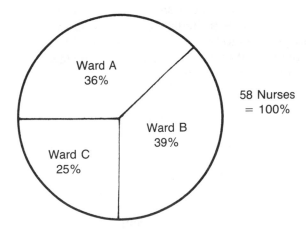

Pie chart showing distribution of staff in surgery unit.

FURTHER READING

Armitage, S. and Rees, C. (1988) Student projects: a practical framework. *Nurse Education Today,* **8** (5): 289–95.

Holm, K. and Llewellyn, J. (1986) *Nursing Research for Nursing Practice.* Philadelphia: W.B. Saunders Co.

Polit, D. F. and Hungler, B. P. (1989) *Essentials of Nursing Research (2nd edition).* Philadelphia: J. P. Lipincott & Co.

7

Examination techniques

As nurse education has moved towards continuous assessment, the emphasis on a single final examination has been removed. This does not mean, however, that you will no longer have to pass examinations but that examinations will only be a part of the total summative assessment for the course. This chapter looks at the various formats of examinations and at how you can prepare yourself to be successful. You should, however, always check the format of examinations with your teacher so that you are aware of what is expected of you.

STATUTORY REQUIREMENTS

The United Kingdom Central Council (UKCC) insists that, in order to meet statutory requirements, colleges of nursing must include a formal written examination in pre-registration courses which will test theoretical knowledge and concepts applied to nursing practice. Colleges are, however, permitted some degree of flexibility in how they plan examinations. This flexibility may mean that you have advance notice of topics, or that you are allowed access to information during examinations. Summative examinations will still include an unseen element so that whilst you may be aware of the topic you will not know the wording of the question. Some colleges still have totally unseen examinations with no prior notification of topic. Regardless of the format of the examination, there are certain factors which colleges must adhere to:

1. All students must take the same examination.
2. Examinations must be invigilated.
3. There must be a predetermined time set for the examination.
4. The specific content of the examination must not be known to students.

The preparation for different styles of examination will differ in some areas and the specific preparation is discussed in the following section.

It should be noted that the UKCC constantly review their assessment guidelines and it looks likely that future assessment schemes may minimize the emphasis on 'examination style' methods. Many colleges are looking at innovative assessments, e.g. interactive programs on computer or video.

PREPARATION FOR EXAMINATIONS

Unseen examinations

If your examination is totally unseen there are several factors you need to identify before commencing your revision programme:

1. What format does the examination take (short answers, essays, etc.)?
2. How long will you have for each question?
3. Are there any revision sessions planned before the examination?

When you have clarified this information you can then plan out a revision programme so that your work is spread out evenly and you do not have to 'cram' at the last minute. When you devise your plan you should work out how many topics you wish to cover and the amount of time you have to work in. You should be able to work out how long you can spend on each topic. Preparing for essay questions is probably best tackled individually and it is useful to look through past papers or make up your own essay questions either individually or in groups to identify the sorts of questions that are likely to arise. Check your practice answers with your teacher.

Mind mapping is a successful way of revising for answering essay questions under examination conditions and Buzan (1989) cites the extraordinary success of students who have accomplished mind mapping techniques. Mind mapping starts from a central theme which branches out with related ideas. Ideas are logically followed through and, by using key **recall** and **creative** words or phrases, the map can be easily remembered.

Buzan defines a key **recall** word or phrase as

> . . . one which funnels into itself a wide range of special images and which, when it is triggered, funnels back on the same image. (p.82)

A key **creative** word is defined by Buzan as

> . . . one which is particularly evocative and image forming . . . A creative word sprays out associations in all directions. (p. 83)

Thus by using a combination of key recall and creative words within a map, you can remember the main points around which you can construct an essay. Examples of mind maps are given on the following pages. Note that the mind maps include numbers to indicate the order of the themes for the essay. The second map also includes pictures which enable you to visualize the themes for the essay.

Mind maps are a useful way of assessing yourself during your preparation period and you can assess yourself in a wider range of material than if you spend time writing lengthy essays. After you have designed your map, you can test yourself by reproducing it from memory and checking it against your master map.

As the examination draws nearer it is useful to write some timed essays. You can either start with a new topic and do a map plus an essay or you can take a map already constructed from your prior revision and write a timed essay from that. Remember that your map has a purpose and you should use it to prioritize points, structure paragraphs and stop yourself wandering away from the subject. It is important to do timed essays so that you can submit them for marking and get feedback on your essay technique and content. If you cannot get a teacher to mark your essay, ask a colleague to look at it for you. If the feedback indicates that you have omitted a theme, add it to your map.

Planning for a short answer questions can be done individually in a similar way but on a smaller scale. It is also useful

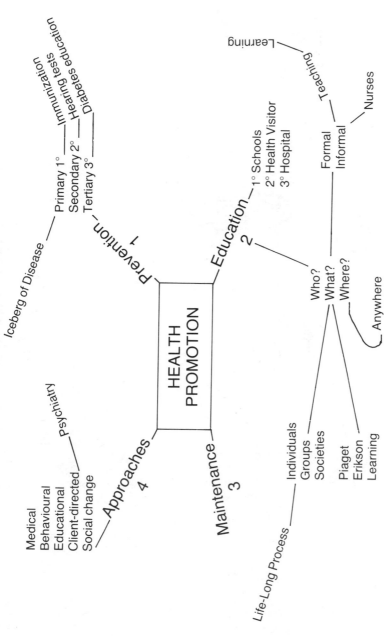

Mind map – health promotion.

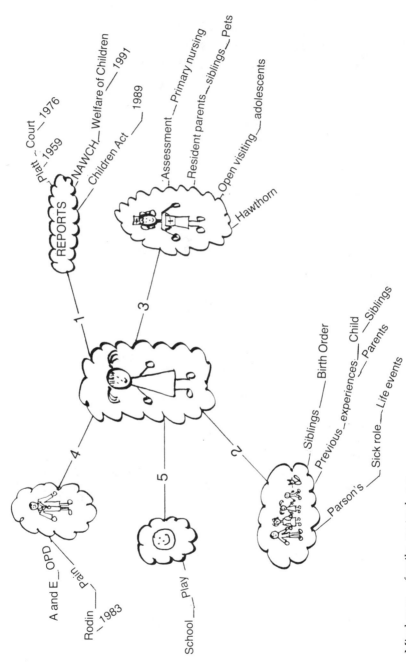

Mind map – family centred care.

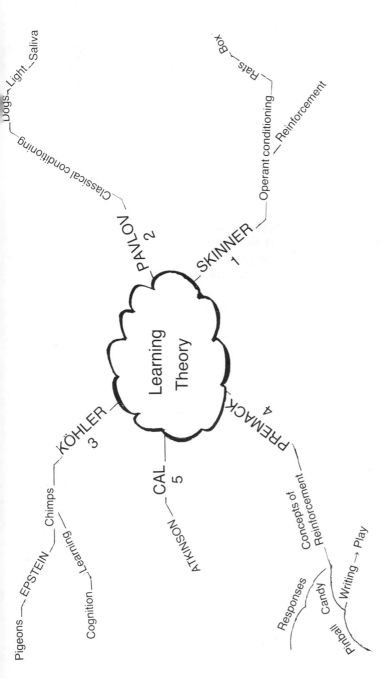

Mind map – learning theory.

to join forces with colleagues and have non-competitive quizzes and joint brain-storming sessions. This is a pleasant and un-stressful way of revising and will give you a break from indi-vidual work. It is also useful for identifying areas that several group members may find confusing and tutorial help on a group basis can then be sought.

Seen topics – unseen questions

Seen topics should in theory narrow down the breadth of subject matter that you need to cover. However, giving seen topics usually means that you will be expected to produce a higher standard of work and show evidence of relevant reading. If you are given four topics and know you have to answer one, you should study one topic in depth but it is a good idea to have a 'banker' topic in case the unseen question for your main topic is totally unrelated to what you have revised.

After you have decided on your main topic and your 'banker', you need to collect your information. You may already have some information in notes and books and you should undertake a literature search (Chapter 2). This will enable you to show evidence of wide reading and you should try to remember author names. It is not usually necessary to remember direct quotations and full bibliographic details. If you can remember the date of the work it is also helpful but not usually essential unless you are referring to a particular report or set of statistics (e.g. the OPCS infant mortality statistics for England and Wales in 1985, the Black Report of 1980, etc.). It is important to remember that teachers can ask you, after the examination, to give the full information on a reference (e.g. the reference about child abuse by Smith).

Although the topic is known, the exact wording of the ques-tion is not and you should therefore try and identify possible questions. The procedure for writing unseen questions then applies, which involves designing a map, writing and then submitting timed questions for marking. A useful way of remembering authors' names is to design your map with the names as your key recall words. (see page 75.)

Accessing literature in the examination

Many colleges allow students to access literature in summative examinations, and students are permitted to take a limited number of books and articles with them. Alternatively, colleges allow students to take a defined amount of notes into the examination, e.g. one side of A4 paper with notes. If you are allowed to use literature you should ensure that you are totally familiar with the material, and in the case of a book you should spend time before the examination using the index as a way of accessing information. There is a great variation in the style and detail of indexes and in an examination it is important that you can access information quickly and efficiently.

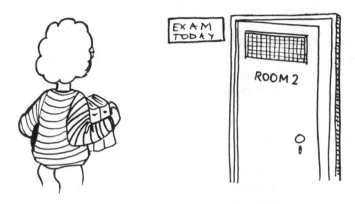

If you are permitted to take brief notes with you, mind maps are an invaluable source of information and they do not take up very much space. It is possible to recall far more information from a map than from written prose. It is also possible to do several mind maps on one piece of paper using different coloured pens – the maps can be written on top of each other and you will still be able to follow them. As with the other forms of examination, try to write some timed answers using your maps and submit them for marking before the examination.

THE EXAMINATION

Few people, regardless of their advance preparation, enter an examination room without feeling at least slightly apprehensive.

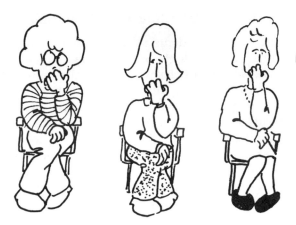

Disciplining yourself to follow a few simple guidelines at the start of the examination can prevent apprehension turning into panic. The following section looks at how to undertake an examination in a systematic and calm way.

1. Turn over the paper and read the question – **twice.**
2. Draw appropriate maps learned during your revision period.
3. **Reread the question**.
4. Check information in the question, e.g. if the question gives you a case history, note relevant points such as the age, marital status and social class of the patient.
5. Make further notes or add numbers to your map to indicate the order of your answer(s).
6. Write yourself a note indicating when you need to finish writing each answer. Allow at least five minutes at the end for reading and correcting spelling and grammatical errors.

Writing your answers

Whilst you are actually writing your answers you should constantly refer to your map so that you do not stray from the question. It is important that you cover a good breadth of material within your question but you should balance breadth with depth. Many colleges award marks for the level of analysis demonstrated as well as for evident knowledge. If you are writing an essay answer, you should also remember to include an introduction and conclusion (Chapter 5).

When you have completed your answer or when you are within five minutes of the end of your allocated time limit, you should carefully read what you have written. Correct any obvious errors and then refer back to your map to ensure you have not forgotten any major points. Ensure that all your pages are numbered and your name or examination number appears on each page.

After the examination

I remember vividly leaving a research examination and walking over to the pub with some of my colleagues. We carefully avoided talking about the examination for the first five minutes and then started to discuss what we had written. I was horrified to realize I had taken a totally different approach to my colleagues and spent the next six weeks convinced I had failed. When the results came I was stunned to find that not only had I passed, but I had been awarded the highest grade of any student in the college since the course had begun!

The moral here is never be tempted to discuss the examination after you have finished. If you are genuinely concerned ask for a tutorial and discuss your worries with your teacher.

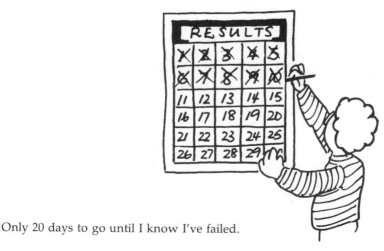

Only 20 days to go until I know I've failed.

PRACTICAL TIPS ON PASSING EXAMINATIONS

1. Carefully plan your programme of preparation.
2. Seek tutorial help if you have any worries before the examination. Most colleges enable you to seek advice and most teachers would rather see you before the examination to sort out your problems than afterwards when it is too late to help you.
3. Try to get a good night's sleep before the examination and have something to eat before you start. Many examinations last for several hours and can be very tiring.
4. Ensure you have a watch so that you can work out your timing for each part of the examination.
5. Make sure you have a pen that you feel comfortable with and a supply of correction materials (if permitted). A few glucose sweets and a packet of tissues are also essential items.
6. After the examination, remember that you cannot change what you have written so try not to worry about failing. Wait for the results which will tell you if you really have anything to worry about.

REFERENCES

Buzan, T. (1989) *Use Your Head* (3rd edition). London: BBC Books.

FURTHER READING

ENB. (1990) *Regulations and Guidelines for the Approval of Institutions and Courses*. London: English National Board for Nursing, Midwifery and Health Visiting.
Rowntree, D. (1988) *Learn How to Study*. London: Macdonald Orbis.

8

Information technology

STEVE HAPPS

Perhaps the greatest advance in the evolution of technology was the invention of the microchip. It has made possible things which only a few years ago were in the realms of science fiction.

For lots of people the thought of dealing with computers fills them with apprehension. However, most of us deal with some form of computer in our daily lives. This may be in the form of a simple pocket calculator or the use of automated banking services. The cash dispensing machine provides a useful example to describe, in basic terms, how computers work and will be used as an illustration later on.

Many people now have access to computers which are capable of performing complex and intricate tasks. The purpose of

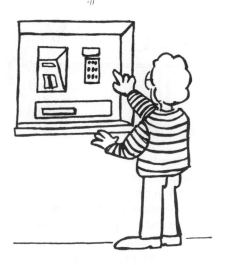

Cash dispensing machines are a form of computer known to us all.

this chapter is not to discuss any particular system or software but how computers can assist in the broad area of study skills.

Technology is advancing at a rapid pace which means that more and more sophisticated products are coming onto the market. Computers today are capable of storing and processing massive amounts of information. To put this into perspective, a standard hard disk on a personal computer can store the equivalent text of up to 50 standard size novels!

COMPUTERS – A BASIC OVERVIEW

One easy way to describe how a computer works is to consider the following simple diagram.

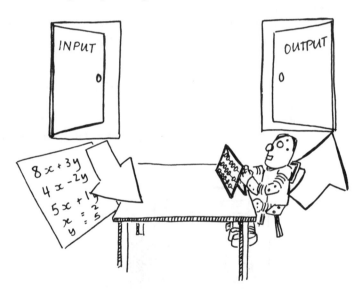

In order to understand, even at a rudimentary level, the function of computers, the notion of data has to be illuminated. Data are information, and in the world of computers this information is digital. Data can be textual, graphic, musical, indeed anything which is capable of producing digital information. Basically the data are composed of a series of binary digits (i.e. 0 or 1) each of which gives rise to the presence or absence of an electrical signal. A series of 8 binary digits is called a **byte**, which becomes a unit of storage capacity. It will hold a number between 0 and 255. These numbers can be used as codes to represent text characters or instructions to the central processing unit (CPU).

Input devices

The most commonly used input device is a keyboard which often resembles a typewriter. It has more keys than a typewriter which allow it to perform special functions. Other examples of input devices are a mouse, digitizer, or joystick; anything which can produce an electronic signal. Think about the cash dispensing machine; the input devices used are your cash card which contains data, and the keyboard from which further data are gained.

Central processing unit (CPU)

This is where the information given to the computer is processed. Programs give instructions to the CPU and tell it how to handle the data given to it. Consider the cash dispensing machine. It requires certain information, some of which is taken from your card and some from your keyboard entry. The machine then performs certain tasks, such as displaying your current balance. The machine itself does not exercise judgement over what to do; it responds to a series of instructions given to it. Basically, those instructions are a complex series of electrical impulses.

Output devices

The two most commonly used output devices are a visual display unit (VDU) and a printer. The VDU is often a monitor but can be a television. There are numerous kinds of printers currently available which offer different qualities of output. The major differentiation is between what are described as impact and non-impact printers.

Impact printers are mainly dot-matrix or daisywheel. The dot-matrix printer is capable of producing characters and graphics formed from a grid of dots produced by wire pins. A daisywheel printer forms characters by a technique similar to that used in a typewriter. The characters (known as 'petals') are mounted radially on a wheel and are struck by a tiny hammer. It produces excellent quality text but is incapable of reproducing complex graphics.

Examples of non-impact printers are laser printers, inkjet and bubble jet printers. These are capable of producing high quality text and graphics.

Other output devices are plotters, speakers, voice synthesizers and robots.

To use our example of the cash dispenser, the output devices involved are the screen, the printer and the mechanical device used to count and dispense the cash.

Memory

In addition to the CPU the computer possesses electronic circuits that store programs and data; in other words, a memory. The two types of memory are Random Access Memory (RAM) and Read Only Memory (ROM).

ROM is used for programs that are used repeatedly and are not modified, such as the operating instructions of a microcomputer or a built-in computer language. RAM holds data and instructions for immediate use by the CPU.

Programs

A program is a sequence of instruction codes that tells the CPU what to do. Since the CPU controls the rest of the machine, a program can access all the available facilities. Programs can be stored in a variety of ways but are mainly kept on disks.

Programs and data are often referred to as 'software', which basically consists of numeric codes given to the computer. On the other hand, 'hardware' relates to all the tangible items involved, for example the keyboard, disks, printer, etc.

Computers can be of great value to you whilst you are studying and they have many uses, the most relevant of which are discussed on the following page.

WORD PROCESSING

Imagine you have been asked to produce a written piece of work for your course. Hours later, after you have finished it, you read it through and decide that it would flow better if you moved some paragraphs around. If you had handwritten this or typed it, you would be faced with a large task. Think of the anguish when you discover it should have been double spaced!

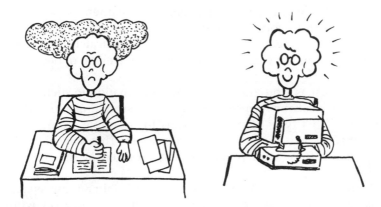

However, if you were using a word processing package these changes would be simple and straightforward. A word processing package is a program which allows for the creation, editing, storing and printing of text. Of course, you still have to type the information in but once this has been done many further amendments and refinements can be made.

One of the great strengths of using a word processor is that it has additional features which allow you to improve on the quality of the finished product before having to print it out.

Most word processing packages allow you to perform such tasks as underlining, creating text in bold, moving or deleting blocks of text, as well as counting words and checking spelling. The advantages to students who have to produce written documents are obvious, as you can save many hours of copying out work which has been done in draft. All these modifications can be done 'on screen', or draft copies can be printed out and discussed. Not only can sections be moved around or grammatical errors corrected, but the whole layout of the document can be changed literally at the push of a button.

Another useful feature of word processing is that other information can be inserted into the text at relevant points. This may take the form of information from within a database program or spreadsheet. One of the strengths of integrated packages is that they make this process much easier.

DATABASE

Imagine that you are writing a lengthy document with lots of references from journals and textbooks. At the end of the document you need to produce an alphabetical list of those references you have used. A database may well be of benefit to you here.

A database is a program that stores information in such a way that it can easily be retrieved by the use of searching and sorting facilities. This type of program can, for example, compile an alphabetical list of references with ease. This can then be imported into a word processor and included at the relevant point.

It could also be used, for example, to maintain a filing system of lecture notes. The program could simply be given a key word (or part of it) and it will then search the data for all relevant entries. Another advantage to the use of a database program is in producing a cross-reference of two or more key items.

GRAPHICS PACKAGES

Consider the piece of work that you have produced using your word processing package, complete with comprehensive references. Within the document are tables of figures relating to the area of investigation. How effective it would be if the figures could be illustrated graphically.

A graphics package allows for the creation and printing of pictures constructed from complex series of tiny dots, allowing virtually anything to be drawn. One of the great advantages to a program such as this is that it can process and display numerical data. This facility is useful when presenting a written piece of work which contains such data. The use of graphics can make dull sets of figures look interesting and can help the reader review the data quickly and easily.

The inclusion of graphics can greatly enhance the overall presentation of a document. However, you must bear in mind that the program will not exercise any judgement over which form of presentation is the best for your purpose.

DESKTOP PUBLISHING (DTP)

This is a program for designing pages of graphics and text as found in magazines, newsletters, adverts, etc. It can produce some visually stimulating results and can be useful for students, especially in producing supporting information for presentations.

The possibilities of DTP packages are endless and there are facilities available for capturing video images or using scanners which scan photographs or other illustrations. However, the costs associated with such items generally render them too expensive for the ordinary user.

SPREADSHEETS

This program is used to store and perform calculations on figures. It is based on a grid of cells using rows and columns. Each cell can contain explanatory text, a number, or a formula that acts upon the contents of other cells. The formulae used can be very detailed and are therefore able to perform some complex procedures. Once a formula has been introduced into the cell then the corresponding figures are produced automatically. However, to obtain meaningful results you must enter the correct formula!

The information stored within these cells can be exported into a graphics facility or a word processing package.

One great strength of spreadsheets is their ability to deal with 'what if' questions which makes them useful in producing forecasts.

STATISTICAL PACKAGES

In addition to spreadsheets there are some packages (for example, MINITAB and SPSS – the Statistical Package for the Social Scientist) which will undertake detailed statistical analyses.

Anyone who has ever been involved in analysing large sets of numerical information will be aware of how time-consuming it can be. These packages can save a great deal of time and frustration, allowing for data to be sorted and processed with ease. It is important, however, that you consider the sort of data you are trying to process. The program cannot make judgements about the characteristics of your data; it just performs whatever task you give to it. Consequently, in relation to inferential statistics, students often make errors when deciding which tests to apply to which data.

COMMUNICATION

This is where data are exchanged between two or more computers. It could be two computers next to each other connected by a lead, or a whole group of networked computers. Going back to the example of the cash dispenser, you can hold an account at one end of the country and yet access information about your account from the other end of the country.

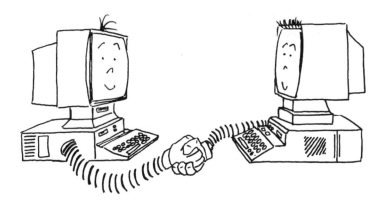

Computers can also be linked via the telephone system using a **modem** (MOdulator/DEModulator). There are ways of reaching a large audience if you require specific information. For example, if you want to find out about a certain nursing technique you could use a computer to access other computer users via, for example, Campus 2000. This would mean that you could have a message stored that other users could read and, if necessary, respond to. Facilities of this kind can be very useful when undertaking research activities.

LITERATURE SEARCH USING COMPUTERS

Imagine that you have been asked to complete an assignment related to a specific nursing activity. One of the first tasks you will need to undertake is a consideration of the literature written about this activity. Once in the library you have to go through index after index, year after year, searching for relevant articles. It would be so much easier if you could access this information 'at the push of a button'.

CDROM

CDROM stands for Compact Disk Read Only Memory. It is similar to an audio CD but is used as a storage medium for programs and data. It is capable of storing massive amounts of information but the computer cannot save information on it, only read from it. It is most useful for distributing large quantities of material that doesn't need to be changed. Many libraries are investing in these as they allow the student to perform literature searches relatively easily. Two commonly used indexes are CINAHL (*Cumulative Index of Nursing and Allied Health Literature*) and *Index Medians*.

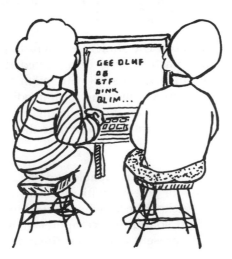

The ability to search in this way allows students to be creative in their searching. In the past the only other options were 'hard copy' searching or 'on-line' searching which usually required the presence of a trained person to retrieve the information.

One other useful facility of the CDROM is that, for some journals, abstracts of the articles can either be read on screen or printed out. This then gives further information in deciding whether or not the article will be relevant to your particular area of investigation.

COMPUTER-ASSISTED LEARNING

During the 1950s B. F. Skinner developed what was known as the 'teaching machine'. The basic notion was to present information to students in a series of frames which could be seen by turning a reel of paper wound onto cylinders. Each frame contained new information and also posed a question for the student to answer.

When computers came along, it was soon realized that devices could be developed which would be far more flexible and responsive than the teaching machine. There are packages now available which give instruction in a variety of areas; for example, basic nursing skills, research, problem solving, decision making.

Computer-assisted learning claims some advantages over more traditional teaching methods.

1. Active participation: The student is interacting with material by responding, practising and being tested at each step.
2. Feedback: The student finds out with minimal delay whether the response is correct, allowing for immediate correction.
3. Individualization of instruction: Students can move ahead at their own rate, and can study at a time that suits them.
4. Revision.

Computer-assisted learning is capable of doing much more than presenting a series of screens with text and graphics. It can manage multimedia experiences where a combination of motion and still video, hi-fi sound and computer generated text and graphics is used to present a learning situation. However, we are perhaps still in the early stages of developing these initiatives.

The English National Board launched the CAL Project in 1988 in order to disseminate throughout the profession the merits of computer-assisted learning. If used properly it can be a useful addition to teachers, but cannot replace them.

COMPUTERS AND NURSING IN THE FUTURE

Nobody can accurately predict the future, but it can be readily assumed that new and exciting innovations will come to fruition. One thing perhaps is clear and that is that technology will not disappear and nurses of the future will require many more skills in this area than their present-day counterparts.

The best way to learn to use a computer is to get your hands on one! Most computers and software packages come with manuals. If you still have difficulty after going through the manual then it is advisable to seek help from an appropriate person. Remember, computers are there to aid you in your quest for knowledge and understanding, not to hinder you.

FURTHER READING

ENB (CAL Project). (1989) Proposal for the Integration of Information Technology to Curricula. Discussion Paper. London: English National Board for Nursing, Midwifery and Health Visiting.

Koch, B. and Rankin, J. (eds.). (1987) *Computers and Their Applications in Nursing*. London: Harper and Row.

9

Copyright

During the course, it is important that ideas, thoughts and information are exchanged and shared with colleagues. However, the Copyright, Designs and Patents Act of 1988 should be adhered to when sharing material which is copyright protected. The Act outlines when copies can be made legitimately and when you could be breaking the law. Parts of the Act are outlined below and a reading list is provided so that you can explore this subject in more depth if you wish.

What material does the Copyright Act protect?

1. Typographical arrangements of published editions. This refers to the whole or any part of published literary, dramatic or musical works, including books, journals, poems, essays, computer programs, songs, etc.
2. Original literary, dramatic, musical and artistic works. This includes graphic works, photographs, maps, paintings, drawings and diagrams.
3. Films, sound recordings, broadcasts or cable programmes.

Who owns copyright?

The owner of copyright is usually the original author, artist, photographer, etc. except where the work was produced as part of someone's duties as an employee, in which case copyright belongs to the employer (subject to any agreement to the contrary).

The owner of the copyright of published editions is usually the publisher. This principle does not, however, apply to Crown or governmental publications.

In the case of a broadcast, the person making the broadcast usually owns copyright, and in the case of a cable programme, it is usually the person or people providing the programme service in which the cable programme is included.

Copyright can, however, be bought, sold or given away.

How long does copyright last?

This depends on which Copyright Act was in force when the work was published (pre-1957, 1957 – 1988, post-1989) and if the work was published when the author was living or dead. The following gives some indication of how long copyright may exist in some instances. However, check before you copy.

1. Literary, dramatic, musical and artistic works are protected for 50 years from the end of the calendar year in which the author died or for at least 50 years from the first publication if the work was not published whilst the author was living.
2. Sound recordings are protected for 50 years from the end of the calendar year in which they were made or from the end of the calendar year in which they were released.
3. Broadcasts are protected for 50 years from the end of the calendar year in which the broadcast was made or from the end of the calendar year in which it was first transmitted. Copyright on repeated broadcasts expires at the same time as that of the original broadcast.
4. Published editions are protected for 25 years from the end of the calendar year in which the first publication of the edition was released.
5. Crown copyright material published prior to 1989 is protected for 50 years after first publication. After 1989, it is protected for 125 years from when it is made or, if commercially published in the first 75 of these years, for 50 years from the year of first publication.

> It is not safe to make assumptions about copyright expiry – check before you copy.

What are you allowed to copy?

1. You can make single copies of copyright material for private study or research provided that not more than a 'reasonable

part' is copied. The Library Association interprets this as follows:

One chapter or extract from books, pamphlets and reports amounting to no more than 5% of the whole work. Up to 10% of a British Standard or two pages if the standard is short.

2. You can make a single copy of a periodical article but not more than one article from the same issue of a periodical. Most libraries ask you to complete a declaration form before you are supplied with a copy or allowed to make a copy.

3. Permission is not needed to make hand or typewritten copies of text or illustrations for research or private study. It is also permissible to copy material onto a blackboard. It is generally accepted that it is permissible to make one overhead transparency or slide of copyright material for the purpose of teaching. However, the Copyright Act does not cover this medium.

4. You may make copies of work which does not indicate who the copyright owner is as long as you have made reasonable attempts to trace the owner. Again, this should be for the purposes of research or private study.

5. You may copy work which is not protected by copyright (usually because a number of years have passed and work is no longer protected or occasionally you will find material which states it is copyright free).

6. You may be able to copy some material if your establishment has a licensing scheme. You need to check the terms of the licence before you copy. If your establishment has a scheme but the work you wish to copy is not covered by it, then there are special conditions which apply which you need to abide by.

7. Educational establishments are allowed to take off-air recordings if the programme forms a part of the curriculum. Recordings cannot be taken of programmes which are covered by a licence, unless the establishment is itself licensed to do so.

8. You may rewrite (but not photocopy) the abstracts of scientific or technical subjects which appear in periodicals.

Infringement of the Copyright

The copying of work is an act restricted by the Copyright Acts. This refers to:

1. Reproducing in any material form, literary, dramatic, musical or artistic work.
2. Copying in relation to a film, television or cable programme, including making photographs from them.
3. Copying in relation to typographical arrangements of published editions.
4. The making of an adaptation of work. This includes adaptations in recorded or written form.

How do you get permission to make copies which are not for private study or research?

The usual practice is to write to the copyright owner asking permission to copy. You should include exact details of which part of the work you wish to copy, how many copies you wish to take and the purpose of taking the copies. It is usual to give assurances that the author will be acknowledged in your work. You must then wait until you have written, signed permission from the copyright owner before copies are taken. It is sensible to keep the original permission reply and if payment is

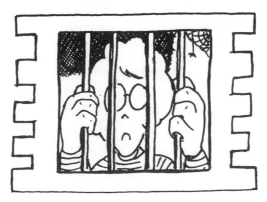

But I only photocopied 2 books!

requested, you should ask for and keep a receipt of payments made.

A final note . . .

Copyright is designed to protect the livelihood of the creators and producers of literary, musical, dramatic and artistic work. Infringing copyright is a breach of the law.

PRACTICAL TIPS ON COPYRIGHT

1. Always 'Think Copyright' before you copy anything. If something is covered by the Copyright Act, adhere to the law.
2. The restrictions on the copying and use of videos and published works are usually clearly stated at the beginning of the video, book or journal.
3. If you wish to ask permission to use material covered by copyright, allow an appropriate amount of time for permission to be granted. For example, if copyright belongs to a publisher in the United Kingdom a month should be long enough, but obtaining permission from other countries takes longer.
4. If you have any doubts about copying all or part of a published work, ask the librarian. Libraries are issued with guidelines relating to the Copyright Act.

FURTHER READING

Crabb, G. (1986) Coping with copyright. *Nursing Times*, **82** (44): 49.
Crabb, G. (1990) *Copyright Clearance – A Practical Guide* (3rd edition). London: National Council for Educational Technology.
The Copyright, Designs and Patents Act 1988. London: HMSO.

Index